Praise for *Boo*

D0979297

"With clarity and compassion, Scritchfield tells us what we desperately need to know: Diet culture pretends to be about health, but actually makes us sick. We end up obsessing over our bodies and forget about our souls. Eating and exercise turn into chores, and self-worth gets dictated by the number on a scale. For anyone who's been poisoned by superficial diet plans and strict food rules, this book is the perfect antidote. Read it if you're ready to stop dieting and start loving yourself and your life!"

—ALAN LEVINOVITZ, PhD, author of *The Gluten Lie*

"It is just not possible to hate yourself to health. *Body Kindness* is a comprehensive, compassionate, and honest user's manual that guides you to nourish, move, care for, and yes, accept your body now."

—MICHELLE MAY, MD, author of *Eat What You Love, Love What You Eat*

"What a pleasure to read such a sensible, self-loving book about improving one's health. Rebecca Scritchfield's *Body Kindness* method honors body diversity—for real! She's not scamming her readers with bogus weight-loss promises. Her weight-neutral, compassionate, and practical approach to health allows people to make joyful, long-lasting changes in their self-care practices."

—CONNIE SOBCZAK, author of *Embody: Learning to Love Your Unique Body (and Quiet That Critical Voice!)* and cofounder, The Body Positive

"Put down that diet book and smash your scale—they don't help you get healthy! Rebecca has taught me that the best thing I could do for my health is to take care of my body and stop fighting it."

—BERNIE SALAZAR, MEd, At-Home Winner, *The Biggest Loser*, Season 5

"If you are ready to stop torturing yourself with diets and self-criticism and start nourishing your body and mind with healthy choices that help you reach your true potential, consider this wonderful book your road map. Scritchfield provides inspiration and real-life strategies in a fun and friendly style, with lots of helpful graphic tools."

—ELLIE KRIEGER, MS, RD, host of *Ellie's Real Good Food* on public television and award-winning cookbook author

"For all of us who've been caught up in punishing cycles of busyness, perfectionism, crazy cleanses, deprivation, too much work, joyless to-do lists, and too little sleep, Rebecca Scritchfield's *Body Kindness* offers a refreshing antidote. In this common sense, warm and eminently practical guide backed by science and story, Scritchfield shows how taking time to pause and set our own internal compasses is the first step toward overcoming deeply held cultural expectations and transforming our lives."

—BRIGID SCHULTE, award-winning journalist and author of the *New York Times* bestselling *Overwhelmed: How to Work, Love, and Play When No One Has the Time*

"Say good-bye to body-shaming and dieting. *Body Kindness* is a refreshing and timely book, which describes how health begins by being kind with self-care actions. Written in a friendly tone (as if you are talking to one of your best girlfriends) by a dietitian who has overcome her own war with her body. Readers will enjoy the stories, infographics, and the many helpful action steps to make peace with food, body, and mind—once and for all!"

—EVELYN TRIBOLE, MS, RD, coauthor of *Intuitive Eating* and *The Intuitive Eating Workbook*

Body Kindness

Transform your health
from the inside out—
and never say diet again.

REBECCA SCRITCHFIELD, RDN

WORKMAN PUBLISHING · NEW YORK

For Audrey and Isla—
May you always see the beauty
in being good to yourself.

Copyright © 2016 by Rebecca Scritchfield

Library of Congress Cataloging-in-Publication Data is available.

ISBN 978-0-7611-8729-5

Design by Jean-Marc Troadec
Infographics by Jean-Marc Troadec, Vaughn Andrews, and James Williamson

Workman books are available at special discounts when purchased in bulk for premiums and sales promotions as well as for fund-raising or educational use. Special editions or book excerpts can also be created to specification. For details, contact the Special Sales Director at the address below, or send an email to specialmarkets@workman.com.

Workman Publishing Co., Inc.
225 Varick Street
New York, NY 10014-4381
workman.com

WORKMAN is a registered trademark of Workman Publishing Co., Inc.

Printed in China

First printing November 2016

10 9 8 7 6 5 4 3 2 1

Contents

Introduction

The Philosophy of Body Kindness

What would you do if you treated your body with kindness?

This is a question I ask my clients, colleagues, friends, family, and anyone else willing to ponder it. I've learned two interesting things from the responses: **Everyone has a gut instinct for how to be kind to their body.** (Nobody says that doing punishing workouts to alleviate cheesecake guilt is a good example of proper self-care.) And quite universally, their responses reflect a deep-seated desire to be happy and healthy, notwithstanding any previous admission that the primary reason they eat their vegetables and go to the gym is to look good.

Most people mistakenly focus on their appearance as evidence of good health (or lack thereof), but looks have very little to do with it. You can be healthy and have cellulite, thick thighs, junk in the trunk, or virtually any body shape. **Health is not just measured physically. Emotional health is an equal part of the equation.** What people really mean when they say they want "health and happiness" is they want to *be well*. The secret to *being* well is treating yourself well and establishing healthful habits you can feel good about.

Creating positive health habits should not drive a person crazy. Yet I am reminded how nutty the health and fitness world can be every time a confused client emails me an article with a title like "Are Eggs Really as Bad for You as Smoking?" Or when a friend tells me they started a new cleanse, are going gluten-free for Lent, or are playing around with Paleo and they want my advice on how to avoid banished foods without looking too ridiculous. In reality, all this rule-following effort is exhausting and unworkable! My friends don't need stealth food-avoidance tactics, what they really need is a Xanax, or better yet, a yoga class or a few deep breaths.

Here's the beautiful truth: You do *not* have to go to extremes to be healthy. In fact, extremes can leave you decidedly unhealthy and unhappy. You don't have to deprive yourself by following diets or "eat clean" lifestyle plans (which are just diets in disguise). You don't have to make big, sweeping changes in your life to someday enjoy better health and happiness. You can have those things right now. All you need to do is practice *body kindness*.

Body kindness is not a set of rules; it's a self-care mindset grounded in the simple belief that health begins by being good to yourself. Through body kindness, you will develop an internal compass for decision-making based on what's actually helpful (as opposed to "good" or "bad"), what you care about most, and the kind of life you want for yourself. The universal body kindness question asks, *Is this helping to create a better life for myself?* The three body kindness pillars can help you navigate this question and serve as guideposts on your journey to better health and happiness:

LOVE. Health grows from love. At the root of body kindness is a willingness to love yourself. Even if you wish you looked different, even if you're having an "I hate my arms, stomach, boobs, thighs, butt, nose, [insert body part here]" day, you can still express self-love in meaningful ways, with every choice you make.

CONNECT. In order for love to thrive, you need to experience an alliance of trust based on connection. You form a bond with yourself, like you would a friend, by being open to observing what your body needs and allowing it to guide your choices.

CARE. In order to build trust, you show your body that you care by making body-kind choices. You express love and connection through caring. It's like telling your body: "We're in this together. I'm your friend, not your enemy."

There's often an uncomfortable moment of self-discovery when a client realizes they really aren't treating their body with kindness. Their facial expression reads like they just saw their kid getting teased at the playground. I can hear their sadness, disgust, and anger as some version of "this sh*t ain't right" passes their lips. For example, I have one client who is obsessed with food rules and believes that she can't possibly enjoy real cookies made with butter and sugar. She needs to make her baked goods "healthy" to make them legal for her to consume. Deep down she knows these dry, flavorless desserts are hardly pleasure-worthy.

Or consider the client whose first instinct coming off a red-eye flight was to head straight to the gym. It didn't matter that she was in a sleep-deprived brain fog, or that work had given her the day off to recuperate. She was bound and determined to burn calories after those big dinners out, and then she was going to catch up on work email before she got back to the office, even if it killed her.

Another client swore she would never be truly happy until she got back to an "acceptable" weight, despite having a loving husband, healthy children, and good friends who loved her just as she was. Even though she was already taking steps to eat well and exercise consistently, it just wasn't good enough. In fact, she'd often skip taking care of herself if it didn't meet her definition of perfect. In our first session, she jokingly said she didn't feel "sexy enough for sex" because her thighs and stomach taunted her during intimate moments. She laughed when she said it, but we both knew she was concealing some pain underneath the humor.

All these women, and many others I've worked with through the years, are plagued by one of the deepest cultural myths of our time: "I'll be happier and healthier when I like what I see in the mirror." For the vast majority of people, this means dieting to lose weight, but it also could mean clinging to a fear of weight gain or feeling the need to alter a body area, like losing a muffin top, shrinking the thighs, or getting a pre-baby body back.

Before I shatter this joyless myth completely, let's take a quick look at what you will gain through the practice of body kindness.

FREEDOM. You are free to make your own choices instead of following meaningless rules. You can stop overthinking and use your energy for interests other than preconceived notions of health and appearance.

PEACE. End the war with your body through acceptance and take committed actions to start living more authentically.

CONFIDENCE. The more you practice body kindness, the more you know you're doing the right thing for you. As the author of your health and happiness, you're empowered to set meaningful goals, even if they don't follow the trends.

Why Body Kindness Works

Body kindness offers a structure for cultivating habits that improve your health without the goal of weight loss. Instead of measuring success in pounds and inches, body kindness is an inside-out transformation. At the heart of body kindness is the art of living consciously. I define this as being present in your life, paying attention to what's happening in the moment (mindfulness), and making decisions that matter to you. A true mind-body connection *and* the equation for behavior change is: HEAD + HEART = HABIT. Your new habits are the result of treating yourself in a way that honors your body rather than punishing it.

As you practice body kindness, you'll learn to integrate compassion, acceptance, gratitude, empathy, and self-worth into your daily life. These are not exactly easy things to do, not even for me, but they are essential elements of the body kindness practice. These touchstones for decision-making will help you navigate through all the wonderful challenges life throws at you while you're trying to change your habits. Using these skills, you can emerge from the normal ups and downs of behavior changes with a belief that you are stronger than you think, you can handle the uncertainty, and you will reach your goals.

Unlike diets or lifestyle plans, body kindness is not intended for people of a certain size or weight category. **Anyone can struggle with body kindness and everyone can practice it.** The following are just a few brave women, representing a variety of weights, shapes, ages, and lifestyles, who have volunteered their story of transformation through body kindness.

Heather

While I did lose weight practicing body kindness, I lost less than I originally had hoped—but I don't even care about that anymore. I learned the expectations I've had for my weight most of my life were unrealistic for my mind and body to truly be happy. I feel like a healthy person now, and I am so much nicer to myself than before. When I see people punishing themselves I feel bad for them because I remember how horrible it was for me. I will never diet again.

Samantha

I sought out body kindness because no other program said it was OK to work on my health without pursuing weight loss, without so-called experts making the assumption that just because I'm fat I must be desperate to change my weight. I made peace with my appearance long ago and used body kindness to build healthful habits I love.

Anna

By looking at me, you would never be able to guess I had an eating disorder. I look healthy. I've completed marathons and triathlons. I'm a personal trainer. People who eat with me assume I eat everything. But the truth is I have struggled on the inside for decades. Body kindness was a framework that helped me save my life and become the person I've always wanted to be.

For many people who have been scarred by diets or body image issues, myself included, body kindness is a way out of the endless on-the-plan, off-the-plan cycle. When you embrace body kindness, you get to ditch anything and everything "diet" because you can't be kind to your body and be on a diet at the same time. You also can't do punishing workouts, body bash yourself, cheat on your sleep, overeat emotionally, drink too much alcohol, let your feelings run roughshod over your health, or do anything else that doesn't fall in line with your definition of being kind to your body. Instead, you'll transform your health through what I call *spiraling up*: Choices that energize you and open you up, like an expanding spiral, and build positive emotions and a strong mindset one decision at a time.

Your brain loves spiraling up because every accomplishment gives it a little reward of the "happy" chemicals dopamine and oxytocin, like tiny high-fives of encouragement. Your mind, body, and heart notice that these things feel good, and you're driven to repeat them. Ultimately, your brain learns and grows from these activities, building the pathways to make healthy, doable choices practically effortless. You'll have more energy, you'll feel better, and you'll create new habits that change your life, once and for all.

People don't always believe me when I say that the best way to build better health is by first making a body kindness choice. Order dessert when you really want it and don't apologize. Give yourself permission to enjoy food in calm, rational ways to avoid emotional eating later. Go to bed on time even though you had hoped to complete more of your tasks that day. After a good night's sleep, you'll have more energy and a fresh brain to accomplish your goals the following day. Schedule a date with friends and laugh your butt off, instead of staying home to balance the bills or catch up on email. Social interaction and laughter are massive mood-boosters that can last for hours, making you more creative and productive. Look in the mirror and tell your body "thank you" for the millions of things it does for you every day without being asked. Self-acceptance is a crucial foundation for freeing up your mind to change the habits that don't serve you. Maybe people are doubtful because this news is delightful, surprising, and pretty much counter to what we are told about self-improvement (no pain, no gain, right?). But it's a fact that is backed by research in positive psychology and behavioral health.

This book will help you practice body kindness through four parts.

....

WHAT YOU DO. Habits like eating, exercise, and sleep choices.

....

HOW YOU FEEL. The thoughts and emotions that influence your day-to-day choices and overall life satisfaction.

....

WHO YOU ARE. Your beliefs and values that help you focus on what's really important to you and why.

....

WHERE YOU BELONG. The relationships every single one of us needs that provide the opportunity to be part of something greater than ourselves.

These parts of the book are parts of you—and they're all important aspects of inside-out transformation.

Through body kindness, you will finally understand how your head and heart can work together to help you live with a deeper sense of satisfaction than you ever thought possible. The real magic of body kindness is that it's completely unique to you, and you don't need to follow any expert's rules in order to reach your goals. If you choose to work with a helping professional, pick someone who respectfully understands that their role is to support and guide you toward a better well-being you desire. Body kindness is not up for other people's judgments. Only *you* truly know if you are being kind to your body in any particular situation. Only *you* will come up with the answers you need to move in the direction you want. And *you* get to reap all the beautiful rewards of creating a better life for yourself.

Why Diets Don't Work

"Can I do a diet first, and then when I lose the weight, I'll do all this stuff with you?" I love when clients have the cojones to ask me this question face-to-face! But after a quick laugh, the answer is always an emphatic, "No."

Before we go any further, let's get clear on diets now, because they're everywhere and you might need something to help you remember that the "six-pack abs program" is about as useful as a space heater in hell. A diet is any plan that promises weight loss as an outcome, usually by attempting to exert control over behaviors, cutting calories, and restricting foods.

Would you take medicine that was proven ineffective 95 percent of the time? That's the failure rate of most traditional diets. Diets are like bad boyfriends. They say, "I love ya, baby!" promising you the world only to leave you broken-hearted. Ironically, when you get frustrated with a lack of results, you give up, blame yourself, and tend to stop taking any actions at all toward better health. Until the next diet comes around, that is, whispering its empty promises in your ear. Then a tiny part of you lights up, hoping "maybe this is *the one*." Psychologically, diets can have addictive properties. Your brain gets a thrill just from imagining reaching your goal weight, and suddenly you're hooked. How else can you explain our sadomasochistic attachment to dieting? On average, a woman will try seven diets in her lifetime (I achieved that goal by eleventh grade). Want to lose weight? Just tube-feed yourself! You won't need any food because you'll be shoving formula down your nostrils! Or better yet, have a device surgically inserted in your stomach so you can drain the food you just ate directly into the toilet. Try the air diet! Just hold your fork to your mouth and *pretend* you're eating. I wish I was kidding, but these are real examples of the dangerous, ridiculous ideas born

from the diet industry. Even diets that may look reasonable to you are nothing but a smoke-and-mirrors illusion creating problems for your mind and body.

In fact, you might as well start calling diets what they are—weight cycling. Because in nearly all cases, weight goes down and then comes back up. A recent study of nearly nine thousand dieters showed that the more a person dieted, the higher their BMI (body mass index) and body weight. Diet once and the odds of weight gain almost double, diet twice and they nearly triple, and **regular dieters had over three times the risk of becoming obese than someone who does not diet**. Not to mention diets' other dirty secrets: Over thirty studies have shown that dieting predicts weight gain, binge eating, and eating disorders. Dieting has also been linked to increased stress, anxiety, preoccupation with food, body image problems, and depression— hardly the components of health and happiness.

Besides their track record of mind and body sabotage, diets are joyless and impersonal. When we follow them we're adhering to other people's rules instead of thinking about what interests us, what piques our curiosity, and what brings us pleasure. These are the very ingredients we need to build realistic and sustainable habits we can live with—or, dare I say, habits we *love*!

DIETS DO MORE HARM THAN GOOD

THE DESTRUCTIVE PATH OF DIETS ON MIND AND BODY

"Ugh...I hate my body. I have to do something."

1. You start a diet, cleanse, challenge, or some other form of food rules, food elimination, and restrained or restrictive eating.

7. You get "hangry" (hungry and angry). You eat richer foods, higher in fats and sugar, and you overeat in reaction to denying yourself nourishment.

6. You produce more ghrelin hormone to intensify hunger signals so you will eat.

8. You feel guilty for overeating. You feel shame about your body. You blame yourself. You continue feeling stressed.

2. You begin to ignore hunger cues. You drink water, eat carrots, or find other ways to "fill up" without really eating.

3. You start thinking about food more often: "When do I get to eat again? What can I eat? What can't I eat?"

5. You produce cortisol (stress hormone) and insulin as the body enters a "food scarcity" mode, signaling the body to store fat and slow metabolism.

4. You feel stressed about your body, weight, and food. You begin to feel more frustrated and hopeless.

9. As your stress continues, so do overeating behaviors and a sense of hopelessness, which set the stage for weight gain outside of your body's natural range.

Still think dieting is the answer to better health & happiness?

DO YOU HAVE A DIETER'S MIND?
Take This Quiz to Find Out.

I try to count calories, carbohydrates, or fat grams as a way of measuring my success around food. **Yes / No**

I use other people's "success stories" as rationale for why I should try the latest diet. **Yes / No**

When I get hungry, I'm hopeful that it's a sign I'm losing weight. **Yes / No**

One of the main reasons I exercise is for weight control. **Yes / No**

When I look at someone else's body, I feel sad (or angry or jealous) about my own. **Yes / No**

If I'm craving a "forbidden food," I usually try to ignore it and make myself eat something healthy. **Yes / No**

I've skipped social events or eaten beforehand to keep my food choices in line. **Yes / No**

I feel guilty if I overeat or eat something I think I shouldn't. **Yes / No**

Answering yes to any of these questions indicates a dieter's way of thinking.

Is There a Healthy Way to Lose Weight?

Hopefully by now you're giving two middle fingers to diets and unrealistic "lifestyle plans" and you're ready to push weight loss goals aside. But I live in the real world, and I understand how deeply people can become entangled in diets, believing that what they are doing is actually in the name of health. I popped the amphetamine-like diet pill Dexatrim like Tic Tacs back in high school (it has since been banned by the FDA). Stroke and heart problems be damned, clearly my greater risk was showing up to homecoming with a few extra pounds (insert sarcasm). Looking back, I feel empathy and sadness for my younger self making poor choices under the guise of "being healthy." I skipped meals to make room for pizza nights. When I felt bad about how I looked or something I ate, I'd assign myself more exercise as penance. At the time I thought this stuff was normal. As a mom, aunt, and friend to mothers of young girls, I hate the thought of people I love doing the things I did, saying the things I said to myself. **If there's a bright side to my suffering, it's that my journey allowed me to find body kindness in myself and use what I've learned to help others disentangle themselves, too.**

If you have weight concerns, you might be wondering if body kindness is right for you. Maybe you still hope that you will lose weight or change your body through this process. For many of my clients, weight loss is important to them. They say things like, "I've got to get this weight off." In some cases, they feel physical pain like backaches and knee problems. Note that people of all sizes can have problems with pain and there may be a cause unrelated to weight. Others recently gained weight related to traumatic life events like the death of a loved one or fertility treatments or another medical condition. Despite my history of struggles with dieting and body image and my firm belief that weight is not a good indicator of health, I still believe there is a healthy way for some people to lose weight. It's pretty simple, actually. Don't set weight loss as a goal—at all. Don't try to manipulate or control your weight. You have to let that idea go if body kindness is really going to take hold and thrive.

When you're focused on weight loss, it's like saying the problem is with your body. But your body is not the problem. Say this three times . . . or a hundred times, until it starts to sink in. When you treat your body like a problem, you carry blame and shame, which results in avoiding behaviors instead of approaching positive changes. It's not your body that needs to get rid of weight, it's your mind. The weight of believing that there is a certain number of pounds you're supposed to weigh in order to be healthy and happy.

Nobody can promise that a specific strategy will lead to long-term weight loss, because all bodies are different—from our genetics to the bacteria colonizing our digestive tract. Our bodies are diverse and are meant to be uniquely shaped. It's simply not true that if you just work hard enough you'll hit a magic number and stay there and be your happiest, healthiest self. But if you absolutely can't take weight off the table, at least commit to practicing body kindness first, and put your energy into transforming your habits. You're more likely to keep weight off if you lose it through realistic and sustainable approaches you can follow for the rest of your life. If your body is meant to weigh less, it should not require drugs, supplements, extreme workouts, or intense self-monitoring to get there.

The Power of the Pen

I suggest treating yourself to a dedicated journal for your body kindness journey. It can be pretty. It can be plain. It just needs to get used. Even if you think journaling is not your thing, approach it with an open mind and give it a try anyway. Writing down thoughts and feelings boosts your awareness of what's happening and why it matters to you, which can be motivating. Writing is a form of self-expression, and you'll be more likely to respond to challenges in helpful ways. You'll be better at planning, generating ideas, setting goals, and tracking important actions. Your mind will become more clear as you spend time getting thoughts on paper rather than letting them buzz around in your head. Having one dedicated place to reflect on your commitments to practicing body kindness is simple and will likely keep you more organized. Think of it as a sacred space for healing.

Make this the first entry in your journal:

The Body Kindness Manifesto

I TAKE CARE of my body every day in ways that are meaningful to me, practicing love, connection, and caring.

DECISIONS THAT ENHANCE my health *and* happiness are best for my well-being.

ALL MY HEALTH efforts, big and small, make a difference in my energy and my mindset.

I DON'T HAVE to change everything in my life right now.

I'M ALLOWED TO struggle and make mistakes in self-care. When I'm having difficulty, I can see it as a challenge and opportunity for growth, not a judgment on my worthiness.

I RESPECT MY body as it is right now, even if I wish I could change it.

NURTURING MY MOST valued relationships and taking time for myself are just as important to my well-being as what I eat and how much I exercise.

No matter what is going on with you right now, know that it's not hopeless and you are not broken. You might be stuck in a place that is no longer serving you, and you're trying to find a way out. You aren't alone. We're each climbing our own mountains, and from where I'm standing on mine, I can see things you can't. Besides me, you have an inner caregiver joining you on this journey. Your inner caregiver intuitively knows how to nurture. She can notice what's happening and help bring a sense of calm and peace while you think about your next step. You can continuously ask yourself, "What would my caregiver do?"

Even if you don't feel it at this moment, you can accept and even love your body. Even if you think you're the worst eater in the world, you haven't exercised in years—or ever!—and you can't name one healthy thing you do, you can achieve better health and happiness. *Body Kindness* is designed to shift your mindset by working with your current beliefs to create new experiences and change how you see things. Once your new way of thinking takes hold and flourishes, you will see the benefits span across your life in unexpected and surprising ways.

There is more than one path to a happy, healthy life. No matter the mistakes of your past, you can always change course.

In Portia Nelson's poem "Autobiography in Five Short Chapters," she tells the story of a person walking down the street who repeatedly falls into a deep hole in the sidewalk and has to fight her way out. Even when she sees the hole is right there, she still falls in. But then, one time, she climbs out as soon as she realizes she's in the same exact place yet again. After that she walks around the deep hole, until one day she walks down another street.

Let's walk down another street together.

"A journey of a thousand miles begins with a single step."

—Lao-tzu

Part One

What You Do

Body Kindness
Is a Choice

Chapter 1

Choosing Body Kindness

The Path to Transforming
Your Health

Philosophy

Each positive choice you make is a little investment in your health and happiness. When you use the power of choice, you can change how you feel in order to influence the next decision you make. Choices have a way of building on one another, giving you more energy to take care of what's important and helping you avoid *choice traps*—situations that can sabotage your decision-making. Body kindness choices should fit your personality and help you feel good. Thankfully, body kindness isn't about making perfect choices all the time. It's about connecting with your body to make loving and caring decisions that eventually take over your life in the form of enjoyable habits.

BODY KINDNESS PILLARS
Make the Choice That Matters Most

LOVE: Do what you love. Choices that fit your interests, personality, and preferences are good choices and they are the best way to express self-love.

CONNECT: Connect to your body. Be flexible enough to change your decisions based on how you feel, what you think your body needs, and what matters to you most.

CARE: Every health choice you make, big and small, is evidence that you care about improving your well-being.

Set Up Your Body Kindness "Comfort Zone"

Think about the term "body kindness" and create your own definition with examples of what it means to you. Use the manifesto on page 12 as a guide to think about the ways in which you want to practice body kindness more consistently.

With your definition in hand, you have a starting point for decision-making.

Now, start tearing down obstacles. Detox yourself from dieting and appearance-focused influences that don't make you feel good or don't help you cultivate a better life. Break up with your old ways and set up a clean slate for body kindness. It's like a colonic for your mind—except this one is free and it works!

Spiral Up

Think about the power of choice. Notice how choices have the potential to lift you up, energize you, and make you feel great. Also notice how some choices don't seem to deliver lasting rewards that are meaningful to you.

The Body Kindness Cleanse

BREAK UP WITH YOUR SCALE. Write a note to your scale, saying something along the lines of "I love myself more than you. You're the manipulative frenemy I never wanted." Tape the note on your scale. Store your scale away. Or skip the letter and take a hammer to your scale. (Stress release is a bonus!) Donating it to Goodwill is another option.

CLEANSE YOURSELF FROM "DIET TALK." This includes conversations with friends and family, and avoiding certain websites, social media, articles, TV shows, etc. Unsubscribe from emails that make you feel bad about yourself and clutter your psyche. Put magazines in the recycling bin or donate them to the nail salon.

PUT AWAY THE DIET PLANS. Trash or donate anything that resembles a weight loss program. Forget about those calorie-counting, low-carb, fat-free diet books. This stuff does not help you be kind to your body. Replace them with recipes and meals you enjoy.

BANISH DIET FOODS. Get rid of anything that has been altered to look like a "health food." Double-fiber cookies, spray butter, those low-carb "miracle noodles" that reek of rotten fish—say good-bye to all of them. Replace them with a variety of wholesome foods you crave.

HIDE YOUR CALORIE TRACKERS. Our accuracy for estimating calorie intake stinks, and it's a major distraction from sensing your body's natural ways of regulating what you eat.

SHIFT ENERGY WITH SAGE SMUDGING. Burning sage—aka smudging—is an ancient practice to get rid of negative energy. You can smudge yourself, your house, your kitchen, or any sacred space that needs to be rid of diet demons. You can also pray, give a blessing, or ask someone to do it for you. These rituals can boost motivation and confidence as you start fresh.

24 HOURS OF HEALTH & HAPPINESS

YOU CAN BE HEALTHIER AND HAPPIER IN JUST ONE DAY

9:30 p.m.
Sleep a solid 8 hours. You'll have energy to tackle the day and prevent food cravings.

7:00 a.m.
Have morning sex. Rise and shine with the "Big O." You'll feel relaxed and in a better mood. (It works if you're by yourself, too!)

8:30 a.m.
Bring lunch and snacks from home. You'll have food you love, nutritious energy at hand, and extra cash!

10:00 a.m.
Refill your water bottle. Every cell needs water. Keep track by adding a rubber band to your cap for every refill. Aim for 6 to 8 a day.

12:00 p.m.
Take a lunch break to enjoy eating without work distractions. Find a comfy space indoors or out, solo or with friends. But no talking about work for the break!

2:00 p.m.
Do a "walk and talk" meeting— it's great for boosting creative energy and your mood.

3:30 p.m.
Afternoon snack attack. If you're hungry, enjoy your snack mindfully, not while racing to meet a deadline.

4:30 p.m.
Take a time-out to re-boot your brain. Take a few deep breaths and name one thing you're grateful for.

5:30 p.m.
Leave work on time. After your "honest eight," it's me time! The work will still be there tomorrow (and on your way out, take a few moments to thank a work colleague).

6:00 p.m.
Get your heart beating. It could be a 10-minute walk, a yoga class, 20 jumping jacks, or a long run. Get some movement into your day before it gets away from you.

7:30 p.m.
Eat dessert after dinner. When you eat "forbidden foods" mindfully, you can avoid eating anything else compulsively.

8:00 p.m.
Do something for pure joy. Plan a vacation. Spend time on a hobby. Give a 30-second hug. Pet your dog.

Make Better Choices Instantly

Saying choices matter feels like I'm stating the obvious. But despite what we may know, we don't always make helpful choices. Just choosing to practice body kindness is already sending you down a more joyful path. Getting started can be as simple as finding opportunities to change, tweak, or tinker with your choice options. When it comes to decision-making leading to habits, the easier the choice, the better. (Your brain is pretty lazy and prefers to conserve its thinking energy.) But you have to find the ways you can work with your brain to make the choices you really want.

Most of the time you know when you're not being kind to your body, because you feel it. Quiet down and listen, and you may hear your inner caregiver. She's probably saying something like, "Hey, it feels pretty crappy when you stay up late binge-watching *Scandal* episodes." But old habits die hard, and you may need some reinforcement to better understand how powerful the simplest choices can be. One way to do this is to ask yourself the universal body kindness question: **"Is this helping to create a better life for myself?"** You don't need a perfect plan to start asking questions and raising your awareness about all the opportunities you have to practice body kindness. The change begins as soon as you start making different choices, and in some cases, it really is that simple for you to be on the body kindness path. Let easy be easy.

Choosing Happiness: The Strongest Way to Healthy Habits

Two mind-blowing happiness facts: *You have much more control over your happiness than you think, and the things you think will make you happier probably won't.* Positive psychology researcher Sonja Lyubomirsky, PhD, has found 40 percent of happiness can be cultivated by daily choices. More money or time, weight loss, youthful looks, and even parenthood or overcoming a major illness have been shown to have little to no long-term effect on happiness in research studies. These life circumstances represent only 10 percent of what makes you happy. The remaining 50 percent is your genetic happiness set point.

These statistics were life-changing for me. When I began to study positive psychology, I was already fully committed in my career to helping people enjoy a better life by building healthful habits, and I thought to myself, "Is it really that simple? Could I help my clients become happier just by helping them make daily choices that would bring them more joy and satisfaction?" On the flip side, I wondered, "Would adopting a healthier lifestyle be quicker, easier, and more effective if my clients were happier?" When I dug further into research, the answer I got was a resounding *YES!* In fact, I figured out that feeling good, being kind to your body, and being happy are all equally important for long-lasting change. Here's why it works:

HAPPY PEOPLE TEND TO VALUE KINDNESS, gratitude, compassion, spirituality, and optimism. This mindset applies both to their relationships with other people and to themselves, increasing the likelihood they will make new habits stick.

HAPPY PEOPLE HAVE MORE POSITIVE EMOTIONS. They notice the "good stuff" when it's happening and they savor it.

HAPPY PEOPLE SET MEANINGFUL GOALS by allowing their values to guide ideas and decisions they feel deeply committed to.

HAPPY PEOPLE ARE MORE RESILIENT. They can bounce back from adversity when it arises and are less likely to sabotage their goals when emotionally distressed.

HAPPY PEOPLE CELEBRATE *IMPROVEMENT* and don't expect perfection. The satisfaction they feel allows them to enjoy the journey as they get even closer to their goals.

Body Kindness Choices Build Upward Spirals

Positive psychology researcher Barbara Fredrickson, PhD, first used the term "upward spiral" as a metaphor for growing happiness, based on evidence that well-being is optimized by gradually building positive emotions one by one, on top of one another. This is similar to the way negative experiences seem to create a downward emotional spiral. For example, a disappointment can make you feel sad and make the workday seem longer, traffic seem worse, and negative feelings multiply, closing you up emotionally and making you feel like you're alone on Woe-Is-Me Island. Fredrickson teaches that upward spirals

Spiral Up

PLAN UPWARD SPIRALS

Open up your journal and draw curved lines in the shape of a funnel or tornado, with the smallest line at the bottom of the page. Each line above it should get bigger, with the largest line at the top of the funnel. Using this design, start at the bottom and write one body kindness decision that makes you feel good. Write down what you do and how you usually feel. Then add another body kindness choice and feeling to it, and so on, going up the spiral. "When I [*self-care choice*], it makes me feel [*emotion*]." Continue all the way up your spiral, building one positive choice and feeling on top of the other. As you start to imagine all this goodness, think about how it impacts other important areas of your life. Write down any phrases that come up in your mind, such as "My creativity comes alive," "I'm more optimistic," or "I'm a better friend." By reflecting on the ways you can spiral up, you will become more aware of opportunities to make choices that are right for you.

can do the opposite. Positive experiences open you up, broaden your perspective, and expand your curiosity as each positive emotion you feel builds on those before it, growing your happiness state.

I believe that you can exponentially grow your health and happiness by layering body kindness choices on one another. The upward spiral you create pulls energy into your life, and your positive thoughts, feelings, and choices fuel one another and keep this powerful energy spiraling up. With this mindset, food, exercise, sleep, downtime, and other decisions are energy giving, not expending. You transfer accrued energy to the people and things you care deeply about and enhance your life in the process, becoming the best version of yourself. If you feel your energy levels depleting, you can make restorative choices.

The beautiful thing about upward spirals is you don't need a lot of time or energy to get them going. You can make a decision—or just have a thought—that grows your upward spiral or changes the trajectory of a downward spiral in an instant. If you get caught in a downward spiral, make the easiest body kindness choice you can think of and start spiraling up again from there. You can literally say, "Wait, this day isn't going the way I wanted it to. What's one small thing I can do right now to be kind to my body?" Then do it. For example, if you're sitting at your desk getting lost on social media when you should be finishing a project, the first step is to catch yourself in the act, and then do one thing that changes the course of your energy. Get up and do ten jumping jacks, pour yourself a glass of water, or just say "Stop, I don't really want this right now." If you're in the midst of a difficult phone call that's making you feel crappy, finish the call while doing laps around the house. If you've already pulled out the ice cream, you can still stop and wait to enjoy it another time when you're not so hotheaded. You'll receive a powerful emotional boost each time you connect to your body and make a choice that is more caring and helpful in the moment.

How do you know when you're in a downward spiral? If you find yourself caught in a pattern of choices that you feel bad about, something isn't right. Check in with your thoughts and feelings. Take a few minutes to rewind your day—without judgment—and notice what happened that led up to your mood. No matter where you are in a downward spiral, the moment you notice what's happening is the best time to flip it upward. I've had daylong downward spirals I didn't notice until right before bed that I tracked back to my first thoughts and feelings of the day. Recognizing that I needed some serious nurturing, I'd pour a cup of tea, write in my journal, take a bath, or do something that felt like a little hug. These choices lead to better feelings, better choices, and better days.

7 Ways to Start Your Day Spiraling Up

What you do first in the day can set your mood, boost your energy, and get that upward spiral going.

If you don't have a morning ritual you love, try one of these seven ideas or create your own. Practice the daily rituals for a month to see for yourself if they help you start—and stay—positive.

1 Strike a "power pose." Stand in front of the mirror, smile, and raise your arms over your head like Wonder Woman. Say something positive like, "I am strong!"

or "I will be kind to my body today!" three times. Change up the poses in between if you feel like it. The book *Presence* by Amy Cuddy, PhD, suggests that the power pose flips a switch in your brain from negative thinking to positive thinking. Your body stances can literally change your mind.

2 **Take some deep breaths.** Find your favorite comfortable spot to sit, then close your eyes. Inhale deeply, allowing your chest and abdomen to expand. Imagine the day's new, fresh sunlight filling each of your cells. As you exhale completely and fully, imagine yourself cleansing within, creating space for whatever the day brings. Release anything from yesterday and prepare for a new day. Focused breathing elicits a relaxation response, impacting your heart, brain, digestive system, and immunity, which is an ideal way to start the day!

3 **Spread gratitude.** Thank your daily helpers—your childcare provider, the bus driver, your barista—for their hard work. Make a new friend while you're in line for coffee. Say good morning to a stranger. Surprise the person behind you by buying his coffee. Human connections make everyone feel good.

4 **Ten minutes of stillness.** Snuggle with your partner or your pet, or just relax by yourself. Breathe calmly and notice things. When you practice directing your mind in a relaxed state, you strengthen your awareness capabilities, which can save you from downward spirals.

5 **Inversion therapy.** Doing a headstand, handstand, or forward bend, or even hanging your head off the side of your bed gives an invigorating, healthy head rush. Get up slowly!

6 **Let the sun shine in.** Eat breakfast by a window or outside for a boost in your brain's serotonin level, which is linked with improved mood. Listen to the birds chirping or other signs of an energetic, living world just outside your door.

7 **Seek to be inspired.** Start each morning with a quote or meditation that sets the tone for your day. The power of our thoughts leads to physical manifestations. Spend a few moments clearly deciding how you wish to shape your day, and then act as if your intention has already come true.

Spiral Up
UPGRADE YOUR CHOICES
TO FIT YOU BETTER

Write a list of body kindness habits and activities, including new ones you would like to form. Do what you think you'll enjoy, not what you think you must do to be healthy or worthy. Some categories to consider are: food and eating habits, fitness, sleep, and fun and leisure time.

For each activity, write at least one benefit it gives you, and write down how you tend to feel about it using one of these phrases:

* It's *natural* and fits my personality.

* It's *enjoyable* and fits my personality.

* It's *important to me even if I'm not enjoying it*. It fits my personality, but I could find other enjoyable activities or ways to make it more enjoyable.

* *I'd feel guilty if I didn't do it.* It's not a good fit for me and not likely to boost my mood or happiness, or to become a habit.

* *I'm doing it to please or impress someone.* It's not a good fit for me and not likely to boost my mood or happiness, or to become a habit.

Put Your Personality into Your Choices

Filling your days with choices that help you experience body kindness through love, connection, and caring for yourself will grow into a life of habits you truly love. One of my favorite things about the freedom from diet rules is that my preferences matter. I get to say what I like and what I don't and I can't be wrong.

Sometimes people feel like the best choice is *always* the healthiest option, but when it comes to body kindness, the best choice is the one that suits you, that motivates and satisfies you. You don't have to settle for anything less.

Body kindness strategies should feel natural and enjoyable and speak to your interests and goals. When you take these things into consideration, you'll care more and try harder to keep up a habit, even when it's not easy.

Using the list of upward spirals you created, **brainstorm how you might step up your pleasure and satisfaction.** Ask yourself: "How can I make this more fun? How can I make sure I do this more often? How can I work around any obstacles that prevent this from becoming a habit?"

Here's one example: You're trying to go to bed an hour earlier to get more sleep, but you find yourself staying up to watch TV. You rated going to bed as *It's important to me even if I'm not enjoying it.* What practical actions can you take that would make it more appealing to turn off the TV and go to bed? Maybe a soothing bedtime ritual like a scented bath, or just making sure you always have something good to read on your bedside table?

If you rated any of the upward spiral activities as *I'm doing it more for someone else*, this deserves a closer look. It's one thing to take care of yourself because you want to be healthy for your children or loved ones. It's another thing to make choices based on trying to please other people. You can use loved ones as positive motivators to keep you going, but forcing yourself to do things because others are nagging you is not your path to body kindness.

By now you should have a list of habits you'd like to enhance or grow, and a sense of how certain choices fit your personality and preferences. Your mission is to let go of choices that don't suit you and replace them with new options that do. Looking over the notes you've made in your journal, create a simple body kindness to-do list based on any ideas you came up with and start putting them into action. **Pick the easiest change and do it first—right now if you can. Early, instant success fuels motivation.** Track your choices for a day or a week. Note how making more feel-good choices impacts your energy levels and mood. You may notice when you track your choices that you're starting to create upward spirals intuitively. Use the information you collect in your journal for inspiring more motivation going forward. You will notice a lot more about what's working and what's not when you're tracking your choices.

Stop, Scan, and Plan

Make more caring choices by *stopping* to notice how much you are (or aren't) enjoying yourself. It might bring about the awareness that you really are experiencing pleasure. Take a second to savor it, and you'll boost your mood! Or you might *stop* and *scan* and notice that you aren't enjoying what you're doing at all. If you're at work and you notice you're taking lots of trips to the candy dish, you might *stop, scan*, and say, "I love chocolate, but I'm not even slowing down to taste it. I'm stressed!" Your *plan* may be "Stop eating the candy, pour a cup of tea, and hold off on sweets until later."

Your Smallest Effort Is Actually a Very Big Deal

Sometimes it feels like our little day-to-day decisions don't make a big difference when it comes to our long-term goals. But if you want to transform the way you think about your health, then every one of these moments represents the beginning of change and the opportunity for pleasant experiences. Looking at your daily decisions through the body kindness lens will create the foundation for your new, lifelong habits. And the littlest decisions should be the easiest to make. "Does this bring me joy?" "What's the body kindness thing to do?" "How can I take better care of myself in this moment?"

The amount of work your brain has to do to make a choice and take action is its *activation energy*. Psychologists recommend you keep the brainpower expenditure low and avoid hemming and hawing over any decision that doesn't have major consequences. You can end up low on activation energy, and then making choices becomes more difficult. If you get stuck, ask yourself, "What's the least I can do?" And do it. Put one carrot on the plate, take a two-minute walk or three deep breaths when you feel emotionally charged. These are the kinds of tiny decisions you can make all day to keep your energy spirals moving in an upward direction. You can always take it further and challenge yourself more. By giving yourself less *mountain* to climb and more *molehill*, your brain will say, "Thank you for not being so difficult today!" and you'll make more body kindness choices.

What do you do when there are choices you know you should make, but you just don't feel like it? Everyone avoids; some people avoid more often than others. It can be a frustrating

Spiral Up
THE LEAST I CAN DO—
30 DAYS OF SMALL, SMART, AND SWIFT

cientists who study behavior changes say consistency is the most important factor for the brain to learn new things. Small efforts are easier to pull off consistently than complicated, time-consuming endeavors. Come up with ten unique and enjoyable ideas for turning this body kindness effort into action (e.g., flavor water with lemon, walk thirty minutes during lunch to clear your head, buy strawberries this week, shut down screens and read before bed). Every idea should be small, smart, and swift. Small because it's easy, smart because you like it, and swift because you'll take immediate action. Go back to the spiral up drawings in your journal for more inspiration.

Put your ideas on a calendar or post your list on the wall and give yourself a daily gold star for hitting your target. Notice the small victories and let yourself feel accomplished.

You'll write your list three times to reach your thirty-day goal. Keep it going until you don't need the reminders anymore. At the end of the month, you may just have one or two new habits from your small, smart, and swift choices!

barrier to creating new habits. I have a couple of mental tricks I use when I have a hard time committing to a self-care decision. Consider how you will feel after you do it versus after you *don't* do it. Another one is to talk yourself into the first five minutes—and then you can quit if it's really that bad. You'll find that the hardest part was getting started, and you're often motivated to finish what you start.

Thalia is probably the most ambivalent and reluctant client I've worked with since starting in private practice ten years ago. When she came to my office for the first time, she was unhappy with her weight and had been binge eating after years of diets. Thalia had experienced some high highs and low lows in her life, from days in the spotlight as a professional opera singer to dark moments of depression when she contemplated ending her life.

Thankfully, with the help of a therapist, Thalia and I worked together to uncover the bright light that years of struggle had buried within her. In fact, against all odds Thalia recovered from binge eating while pursuing a PhD and working full-time. Over a two-year period, we discovered that she had undiagnosed ADHD, which took a significant toll on her confidence and her ability to follow through with healthful choices.

Thalia could easily get tripped up when it came to all the details of grocery shopping, meal planning, and food preparation. She needed help setting simple, realistic goals and following through on them. She also needed to build self-compassion. She was so nasty to herself—always criticizing, bullying, and shaming. Any small success was met with a sharp "not good enough" retort. Thalia often struggled with the downward spiral effect of poor choices. Staying up late to unwind in front of the TV led to poor sleep, which led to being tired, which led to skipping the workout (if it had even been planned) and saying "screw it, let's get pizza for lunch!" There were times I thought she was going to give up and walk away. But she never did, and I took it as a sign she was much stronger than she gave herself credit for.

Thalia's first big upward spiral came when we set the modest goal of fifteen minutes a day of joyful movement—it didn't matter what kind of movement, any movement would count as having met the goal for that day, whether it was a few laps in the pool or a stroll around the block. By freeing herself from all the heavy expectations of her past, Thalia began to realize she had many reasons to loathe exercise. It was how she punished herself for poor eating. And it was what she did to try to change her body, not take care of it. The turning point came when she began to see these negative thoughts and feelings as self-sabotaging beliefs she needed to walk away from. Being kind to her body meant these misguided "motivations" for exercise would be part of her past, not her destiny. Finally, she could let go of self-defeating behaviors and take back control of her life with small, consistent choices that were important to her.

Inspired by the success of this approach, Thalia's next small step was getting back into yoga. But this one held a lot of emotional turmoil for Thalia, and it wasn't easy to overcome the mean voice in her head saying, "You had a great practice ten years ago; now look at you." Determined to remain open to opportunities for growth, she finally said "just this *one* class." The instructor was very encouraging and invited her to a class the next day, and Thalia went! Thalia had known all along that her choices matter. She needed to say yes to one small choice and experience the upward spirals that resulted. There have been bumps in the road and setbacks along the way, but now Thalia knows that when a challenge arises she just has to do the next right thing and she will keep moving in the right direction.

Choice Traps

Personally, I have to fight the urge to jealously rage at anyone who makes choices and actions look easy while I'm hard at work trying to make things happen. The simple truth is that having knowledge of what you need to do is not enough to actually do it, let alone turn it into a habit. You also need to *believe* your effort can make a difference, and unfortunately many people are their own worst enemies when it comes to turning choices into action. I call the mental and emotional hurdles we put ourselves through *choice traps*.

Choice traps are like booby traps for your good intentions. They are the impulsive and irrational mindsets that make healthy decision-making unnecessarily difficult. Choice traps fail the universal body kindness question and ignite downward spirals, and most of the time we don't even know it's happening. Here are four choice traps to avoid.

CHOICE TRAP #1:
HERD MENTALITY

Human beings are herd animals. We survived only because we clustered together in herds, like other animals, to share resources. Our brains have not evolved enough to make it easy for us to ignore what everyone else is doing and focus on what we want. When our pack is going down a path, we're going, too, even if it leads nowhere good. We don't want to be left out. In the days of cavemen and cavewomen, staying in a group meant survival: food, safety, and sex. In today's times, we deal with the fear of missing out—FOMO. "She's all excited about this new diet. I should do it, too." (I'll be the only one who can't fit into my bathing suit on vacation.) This is called social comparison—we make up stories about how great other people's lives must be and use them to judge ourselves and put ourselves down. I lovingly refer to this concept as *compare and despair*. FOMO and social comparison can lead to irrational, misguided decision-making fueled by fear and competition to fit in. The sneakiest part about this choice trap is that it causes us to make fear-based choices instead of feel-good choices without even realizing it!

The first step to overcoming herd mentality is to acknowledge what's going on and run it through your body kindness filter. Ask yourself, "Is this really what I want or is this FOMO?" Remember the "F" in FOMO means "fear"—a feeling that does not help you make rational decisions. Think about whether or not the choice will still matter to you in a year. Maybe it *is* something you really care about. Consider sacrifices you may need to make to follow the herd. Is it worth it? Make sure your choices are rational and they reflect what matters to you, leading to upward spirals. Follow your inner caregiver, not your neighbor.

CHOICE TRAP #2:
MORAL JUDGMENTS

Choice-making is an inside job. Maybe you have a friend who chokes down a shot of apple cider vinegar every morning, and you prefer your vinegar with french fries. She may run marathons and you're more of a Jazzercise kinda girl. Does this make either one of you a better or healthier person? Of course not.

Sometimes we need reminding that our personal choices have nothing to do with moral character. Besides the fact that slinging verbal vitriol at ourselves serves no real purpose or benefit, there's another important reason you should avoid any moral judgment around choices: Anything you moralize leaves you susceptible to a little psychological phenomenon called *moral licensing*, where *being good* unleashes your urge to *be bad*. You may use completely irrational logic to justify a behavior: "I was so good at this workout, I deserve the chocolate cake." Or the reverse: "I didn't earn this dessert, so I deserve to suffer and go without." Labeling behaviors as good and bad can lead to obsessive self-monitoring and shaming. Watching your every move tires out your brain and eventually unfurls a part of you that does not want to be controlled. You give yourself something to rebel against every time you lay down an inflexible, moral law. I don't like to be controlled—do you? The power of choice is a freedom our minds don't give up easily.

Counterintuitively, the more we try to control ourselves in rigid ways, the less self-control we have in the long run.

Instead of unleashing moral judgments, practice body kindness by making choices that matter to you. Be flexible with your options. Don't look for rewards every time you do something virtuous and punish yourself when you don't. **The best choices you can make don't need any more reward than the satisfaction you feel after making them.** Reflect on how your efforts are contributing to your goals. Share your excitement with others. You might inspire them, or at least you'll get the reward of shared joy. Give yourself a mini, meaningful reward if that motivates you to keep going. Choose something that strengthens your commitment to yourself and helps you feel good in the moment, for example, a new workout top or exercise headband, a new kitchen gadget or a massage.

CHOICE TRAP #3:
IMPULSE DILEMMA

Do you ever feel like there's a devilish saboteur sitting on your shoulder who commandeers your brain during micro-moments of decision-making? When you hear yourself saying "Oh, that's tempting," you're in the presence of an impulse, and this can make you feel like you're Superman staring at a pile of kryptonite.

One way to keep your self-control in check, even when you're distracted by your impulses, is by taking a deep breath and bringing your attention to your options. What happens if you pause and think about your options—not just your instinct? Imagine holding the two opposing choices in your hands at the same time. In one hand, there's the easier choice you feel compelled to make (veg out in front of the TV for a few hours before bed). That's your immediate reward. In the other hand is the harder choice, but it's usually the one that matters to you more. (Go to bed now. You don't want to drag your exhausted self around all day tomorrow.) The second choice offers a more distant yet more satisfying reward. Here's the kicker: You get a dose of pleasure just from making a decision. If you find yourself with two seemingly opposite choice options, slow it down and think rationally. Which one of the two do you care about more? Which one helps you create a better life and spirals you up?

CHOICE TRAP #4:
CHOICE OVERLOAD

You just need to think about the number of options we have for yogurt, bread, and eggs at the grocery store these days to understand that we have too many choices to make in most areas of our lives. The stress you feel from trying to make the best choice from an array of too many options reduces the satisfaction you're supposed to get from choosing in the first place. You take longer to decide while you compare options—"Hmm. This yogurt has 13 grams of protein and 2 extra grams of sugar. But the sugar is from fruit, so maybe that's OK. But this one is on sale and it's organic." And then there are all the flavor varieties. Once you finally choose, if you're not mentally exhausted and racing to the candy aisle for a Kit Kat bar to quell your emotional overwhelmedness, you might be questioning whether your choice was really the best and actually feeling *bad* about it like you somehow could have done better.

Avoid *choice overload* by refusing to play the game. Don't dawdle. For simple choices, such as grocery items, research shows we have about thirty seconds before we start confusing ourselves. Save your brainpower and emotional energy for more important things in life. Don't stress over broccoli versus cauliflower. Get a vegetable and move on. See the chance to try new brands and flavors as an adventurous experiment, not the be-all and end-all. Make it your goal to become great at making good enough choices whenever possible. You'll be happier (and healthier) for it.

Another way to avoid choice overload is to give yourself routines so you won't have to waste time overthinking: Make 80 percent of your shopping list good foods you always buy, set recurring appointments on your calendar for some type of exercise, and plan what you'll do later. Go to bed at the same time, and don't get distracted by your television or smartphone.

Committed Actions Create Habits

Until your behavior is a consistent and relatively effortless habit, it can feel like you're wasting energy piecing together choices like a second grader's papier-mâché art project. Things can get messy, so I encourage you to take a closer look at your motivation (or lack thereof) to help clarify why you're making certain choices in the first place. If you feel like you're practically forcing yourself in one direction, usually out of external pressure, you might be struggling with misplaced motivation, ambivalence, or lack of clarity on what you really want.

One of the least satisfying reasons for change is following what someone else is pushing you to do. We know how that goes: The more others give you reasons to make a change, the more likely you'll find reasons to stay the same. Try as they might to "influence" you, they only push you further away and distract you from making positive changes you may want for yourself. Your brain builds up resistant thoughts that can sabotage your efforts. You begin to wonder what's wrong with your motivation. Why are they more excited about you making a change than you are? In this situation, you need to put motivation back in its rightful place—with you.

Intrinsic motivation, the kind that comes from within, is more likely to lead to long-term habits because it's built on your curiosity, interests, and desires. When making choices, ask yourself, "What do I want to do?" If something is important to them and not you—tough cardboard cookies! Just be you. Any choice you make for yourself in the name of body kindness is the right choice. You are in charge and accountable for your actions. Sure, you can invite others to help support you and hold you accountable to your goals. You can even look to others for inspiration and encouragement! Just remember that you're in control here. You're driving the car. You decide the speed, control the gas pedal and brakes, and choose the roads you take on your journey.

Low intrinsic motivation brings about another choice trap—ambivalence. Wanting to make a change and not wanting to at the same time is one of the most deeply embedded mindsets that can undermine success. You could have all the reasons to make a change, all the resources you need, but you just can't find the will to keep moving forward. You might make some choices that support behavior change, but nothing consistent enough to push you past ambivalence. Maybe you give yourself a hard time, saying things like, "You're never going to change" (or some other type of failure message). This fixed mindset—when

Spiral Up
TALK YOURSELF INTO CHANGE, *DARN* IT

Use the handy acronym DARN to get clear on what you want and the choices that will help get you there:

* **Desire:** What do you hope to accomplish? Take ownership of what is important to you. Think about what would bring you pleasure, joy, and happiness.

* **Ability:** How likely is it that you will be able to accomplish it? Use a scale of 1 to 10. The higher your confidence, the better. If it's on the low side, ask yourself, "What would it take to get to a higher number?"

* **Reasons:** What might be good about accomplishing your desire? When you think about the benefits, you're building an emotional connection to your ideas and accelerating your intrinsic motivation.

* **Need:** What needs to happen? Here is where you come up with your creative ideas for accomplishment. Identify resources you need to procure, or other choices you need to make, such as a shift in priorities.

you don't believe change is possible—is a self-fulfilling prophecy.

Here's the good news: Ambivalence is a normal part of the change process and the most common place to get stuck. What a relief, right? A little self-compassion can go a long way. Agonizing or judging yourself for inaction doesn't motivate you to move forward with the confidence you need to succeed. The trick is to build up more reasons to change than not to change. One small healthful choice at a time, you can push past ambivalence and string together choices you feel good about. You can do that by talking yourself into it. (I'm serious.) Get excited about change with the DARN IT activity.

"I Have No Motivation Mojo"

Many people who have difficulty changing a habit see their struggle as a sign of weakness. In their effort to avoid stress, they may feel like giving up. Two of the primary reasons for quitting a healthy behavior change are lack of enjoyment and absence of immediate rewards. But accepting that challenges are a normal part of the process and having a willingness to engage with difficulty are signs of strength. When you are faced with a challenge, obstacle, or difficulty, it triggers a stress response in your body and results in an outpouring of energy. How you use that energy is up to you. Remember: You want to work on the body kindness goals you set. You want the benefits of that new habit you're trying to form. It might sound cliché to say "believe in yourself," but you really do need to believe that you have the ability to form new habits. You also need to give your brain a chance to learn and grow.

Think of learning as a constructive process rather than a chore. If you were teaching a child to ride a bike and he or she fell off, would you toss the bike in the trash? Absolutely not! You would help, coach, and provide encouragement. Think of your effort as a sign of your resilience, not your shortcomings. Each time you fall, consider it a chance to prove you can get back up.

When finding your motivation feels impossible, grab on to any glimmer of hope you can and identify one good choice within your reach. Hope is not just a wish. Hope is the will *and* the way. **Having hope boosts confidence, and when you are confident you can handle a change that is important to you, your internal motivation is at its highest.** Short on hope? You can cultivate some by looking back at any past successes or achievements you experienced, no matter how little they may seem right now. If you're really struggling, perhaps the best thing you can do is notice that your hope and confidence are lower than you would like them to be. When you feel like quitting, you could say, "Well that's no surprise because this is difficult. I'm working on growing my confidence." Continue to encourage yourself and eventually you will talk yourself into change.

Choose to Put Yourself First

I have one foolproof strategy for strengthening your well-being and avoiding all of the choice traps: Choose to put yourself first! This is the most important choice you can make for yourself and everyone you love. Your efforts to practice body kindness must come ahead of your job, family, closest friends, spouse, partner, and children. Is that hard to hear? I know when I imagine putting my needs ahead of my kids', my heart aches. But look deeper. You need to do this because you love others so much. If self-care isn't highest on your to-do list, you will deplete your energy and spiral downward. You will have difficulty focusing, staying positive, and being happy. Everything else in your life suffers when you don't put yourself first.

One of my nutrition mentors, Evelyn Tribole, once told me, "Rebecca, you can only take people as far as *you* have come." Her statement was so potent, it has become the foundation for everything I do at work and at home. How can I possibly be the best version of myself without consistently, repeatedly, and unapologetically putting *me* first? This realization inspired me to create an intervention of sorts for clients who have difficulty embracing this "me first" philosophy. I purchased an airplane oxygen mask online, and I ask clients to hold it in their hands and repeat the phrase they know well but don't do. "Secure *your* mask before helping others."

I never could have guessed how often this simple exercise would bring even my most composed clients to tears. They cry because they know it's true, no matter how difficult it seems. They painfully recount when time and time again they put their self-care on the back burner. They feel the downward spiral of energy and mood all over again in my office chair. "Me first" is probably the most important and most difficult choice you will make on your body kindness journey. Anyone who is part of your life will learn from your example. This is a priceless gift you can give them. In order to be the best person, mother, teacher, sister, employee, or friend you can be, you have to put yourself first, even when it feels difficult to do so.

- -

BODY KINDNESS REFLECTION: Spend fifteen minutes journaling your thoughts and feelings about how the power of choice can help you have a more joyful, healthy life.

- -

"Everything can be taken
from a man but one thing:
the last of the human freedoms—
to choose one's attitude in any
given set of circumstances,
to choose one's own way."

—Viktor E. Frankl,
MAN'S SEARCH FOR MEANING

Chapter 2

Eating with Body Kindness

Free Yourself from Food Rules

Philosophy

The art of eating well encompasses much more than the nutritional value of the food that ends up on your plate. Your food traditions, food preferences, and social calendar all play a vital role in influencing your food choices. Eating has the potential to be a trustful, intimate connection between you and your body. But if you're stuck in a rigid framework of rules that dictate your food choices, you're probably missing out on some meaningful opportunities to enjoy a variety of foods in healthy, guilt-free ways. Instead of narrowly viewing food choices as a matter of "good" vs. "bad," practicing body kindness will help you explore new, flexible ways of thinking about food and encourage you to consider the positive role that food can play in your well-being.

BODY KINDNESS PILLARS
Aligning Food Choices
with Body Kindness

LOVE: Choose foods you love to eat and unapologetically leave the judgments behind.

CONNECT: Respect your body's communication signals for when and how much to eat, regardless of what's on your plate.

CARE: Instead of striving for perfection, allow your eating patterns to strengthen your confidence as your body's competent caregiver.

Be Flexible with Food Choices

How many food choices do you think you'll make today? Brian Wansink, PhD, director at the Cornell University Food and Brand Lab, found that, on average, people make over two hundred decisions about food every single day. No wonder it can get confusing—overwhelming even. But look at the bright side: With all these opportunities, there's room for flexibility. Trying new foods and enjoying our favorites—that includes some "junk food"—are part of the joys of life. "Wait, did the nutrition expert just give me carte blanche for *all* my food choices?" In a way, yes, I did. Freedom feels great, doesn't it?

When you embrace body kindness, you don't need food rules to guide your choices. You have your preferences, your standards of what matters to you, and your wonderful "body signals" to guide your decisions. Instead of thou-shall-not-eat lists, you just need a workable solution that helps you eat in life-enhancing ways. Food choices should spiral you up in energy and make you feel good physically and emotionally. I've created a very simple, straightforward guide to help you make your food choices. My approach has only three parts, with room for flexibility, giving you options instead of rules.

Spiral Up

Think about a recent joyful food experience. What did you eat, where were you, who were you with? What are the different ways your food choices can be a form of body kindness? How does lack of confidence around making food choices get in your way of practicing body kindness?

1: Be hungry. 2: Balance your plate. 3: Savor your meal.

This body kindness guide for making food choices offers a structure that many people are looking for after breaking up with their "bad boyfriend" diets. **You no longer have to waste valuable brainpower overthinking what, when, how, and why you should eat.**

I like a three-legged stool metaphor because it shows just how important balance is when you want to feel your best and take care of your body. The stool functions when all three legs are working together, all vitally important, all doing their share of the work. There are many ways you can grow your body kindness practice using this three-legged stool for eating well—and remarkably, none of them involve crazy food rules! But before I start showing all the goods, I'm going to ask you to open yourself up. If you are really nervous about swapping out fear-based food rules for your food preferences, you probably think something terrible is going to happen if you start eating banned foods again. But everything changes when you begin to allow mindfulness and calm, rational thinking to guide your food choices. I'll help you understand why rules are the main culprit for your lack of trust around food and I'll give you some body kindness tools to set yourself free.

Explore Your Food Preferences First

When was the last time you put good thought into *why* you eat what you eat? Do you focus on taste, convenience, cost, quality, and health benefits? As with most areas of life, enjoyment drives your food choices. It's natural to crave taste bud-pleasing foods and to avoid unpleasant ones. In fact, your "ick factor" is what keeps you from eating moldy food and drinking spoiled milk—thankfully.

No matter what drives your choices, there are countless ways to find a good fit for you and your family. The one thing there is not room for is fear. If thinking about food leaves you feeling guilty, anxious, or afraid, you probably have a problem with unnecessary food rules. (More to come on that later.) First, let's just put aside any judgments about food, including what's "healthy" and "unhealthy." Later on I will show you how to boost the nutritional power of virtually any meal with flavor tips, ingredient swaps, and balanced plate strategies.

Open up your journal to a new page and write the heading *What I Like to Eat*. Be honest here. No matter what you write down, it's OK, as long as it's truthful. **Think about foods that bring you pleasure.** Brainstorm what you would like to enjoy at a celebration, on vacation, or at a summer barbecue. Name your favorite restaurant dishes and types of cuisine. Think about what foods you like to prepare and what feels good in your body. What are your most favorite things to purchase at the grocery store? What do you look forward to eating throughout the seasons? Do you have any favorite food memories? What comfort foods make you feel like you're getting a nice, warm hug? Pretend you're a food writer and describe why you like these foods with some detail. Hopefully you're salivating just thinking about food you love. If you notice any judgmental thoughts coming up, try to let them pass and just keep writing until you think you have adequately described the foods that bring you joy.

When I do this exercise with clients, it can be a very challenging experience. Some clients are uncomfortable admitting to me that they truly love pork rinds or McDonald's ice cream cones and their mind is flooded with thoughts like, "Oh, you're terrible. That's soooo baaaad." Other clients struggle because they simply don't know what they like anymore. They just know they are tired of broiled chicken breast with steamed spinach. Many people have been brainwashed to look for rules for what they *should* enjoy as opposed to deciding what they *actually* enjoy. But guess what? The human body was not invented yesterday. Satiety, the natural feeling of fullness that signals the time to stop eating, is partly determined by the enjoyment of eating. Putting food you want to eat on the plate in the first place is essential in helping your body figure out how much food to consume.

If you're thinking, "But what about the unhealthy food I overeat; it can't be good for me." I have two responses: **What if the reason you overeat is because you don't let yourself enjoy it often enough?** Like a one-day sale at Macy's, you need to act now and max out your credit card with all the great deals before the sale ends. Tick-tock. When you finally give yourself permission to eat foods that really taste good, your brain has learned this won't last long, and then it's back to chicken and spinach. So like an anxious Macy's shopper, you go a little overboard. Or what if the reason you choose to eat certain foods is for emotional hunger and not physical? Your brain also learns, "When I'm sad, I eat chocolate dipped in peanut butter." If that's something you really like to eat, the trick is to disassociate specific food choices from soothing specific emotions. (Much more on that later.) For now, trust that nobody is going to judge you for writing down foods you like to eat in your journal.

There are ways to balance out your taste preferences and your desire to nourish your body—from choosing how you prepare food to how you eat it. One of the most interesting insights I have seen in my clients and my own food liberation is how some foods suddenly lose their irresistible allure when you stop avoiding them altogether.

It's one thing to avoid foods because you don't like them or want to change how you eat a food. I wouldn't argue with a person who said, "When I eat chips, it's usually out of the family-size bag while watching TV at midnight and I eat too much." But I have witnessed some of the most absurd food rules as of late. Here are some of the ridiculous things I've heard: "Don't eat anything white." "Potatoes are fattening." "Corn is too high in carbs." "I'm avoiding carrots because of the sugar." "I eat fruit only with a protein." Hello! What? Only 11 percent of Americans get the recommended amount of fruits or vegetables a day. We should be eating more produce, not talking about eliminating nutritious potatoes, corn, and carrots.

Are Food Choices Driving You Crazy?

Many of my clients feel overwhelmed by all the conflicting advice on what to eat. These days it's not enough to simply eat produce; there's an all-out war going on over which cucumber, carrot, or melon is "the best" for you. I'm going to give you a free pass, and ask you to let go of the "buy only organic, GMO-free, farmers' market" agenda for the time being. Here's why: You don't have to pick a side to practice body kindness. You just need to feel good about taking care of yourself and aligning your personal food preferences with your budget and time constraints. As you are trying to build new habits, the last thing you need to worry about is trying to outsmart the food-marketing experts! Take conventional vs. organic. The food companies are going to make whatever people will buy. Some companies produce both organic and non-organic varieties of produce because there is a market for both. You win eating any fruit or vegetable (even the starchy potatoes and sugary strawberries have nutrients) so I suggest keeping the internal debates on which is best to a minimum, at least until you have already become a person who regularly fills her plate with all the colors in the rainbow. It's also worth mentioning that, as of this printing, scientists have not found any discernable differences in the nutritional content of organic vs. non-organic produce. And in May 2016, the National Academy of Sciences released a 400-page report declaring GMO foods just as safe as non-GMO foods. So, what should you do? Buy food that fits your personal taste and budget. Don't stress!

Only you can decide what makes you feel good. Some people just know what they want to do; they have a nice-sized grocery budget and it's easy enough for them to look for organic. But others are stretching their dollars, just trying to cook more instead of taking the more costly and easier approach of ordering

delivery. Still others would be happy if their family just said "I will eat broccoli!" **Most people are simply confused and want someone to tell them what to do.** In this scenario, I'm Switzerland. I'm totally neutral. If someone you know is really passionate about eating only organic or GMO-free, it doesn't mean you have to be, too (remember "herd mentality" and FOMO). Especially if deciding what to buy and eat causes anxiety—that's probably worse for your health than anything you're eating. Virtually anything can be made with organic ingredients, even Oreos, but just because it has a green leaf on the label or a stamp of approval doesn't automatically mean it's good for you. Choose to see the bright side. You have choices and you really can't mess it up, especially when debating the health merits of organic and conventional produce, yogurts, and peanut butter.

I've read enough biased news stories from both sides over the years to motivate me to stay focused on the bigger picture. First and foremost, the food industry is responsible for adhering to practices that produce safe food and prevent food-borne illnesses. I'm grateful to have access to safe and affordable food year-round. I choose to care most about respecting individual preferences and choices. Your preferences are yours, and they aren't up for anyone else's judgments. You can still wear the "I care about what I eat" T-shirt even if you buy the non-organic blueberries or the artificially flavored coffee creamer. Your food preferences do not have to be whittled down to a short list of unexciting, "clean" produce. Flexibility and moderation may not be sexy sales-driving messages, but they are the very essence of building long-term habits and lifelong happiness, so it's about time we cut ourselves some slack. When your food choices feel good to you, trust that you are practicing body kindness your way.

Food Rules Are Sabotaging Your Best Intentions

"I want to be a normal eater" is the most common food-related wish I hear from clients. For anyone who has been "at war" with food, the mere thought of eating can be a source of overwhelming stress and anxiety. Instead of a positive connection with food, there's fear. Maybe you use food to numb or escape painful feelings. Maybe you worry over what you should eat, cling to rigid food rules, or even avoid social events when food is present. Food can be your best friend, evoking wonderful memories, or your worst enemy, filling you with anxiety and self-doubt. The biggest difference between a food preference and a food rule is a very powerful, little four-letter word: *F-E-A-R*.

Food, as a general rule, is not toxic, but the fear of food can be. Our culture has developed an obsession with pure, clean, and otherwise "perfect" styles of eating, to the point where food isn't even food anymore; it's a judgment.

Self-flagellation has hijacked the joy from our everyday life and special occasions. Food is either good (kale) or bad (cupcakes). We are morally good or bad people based on our food choices.

The pressure to be hypervigilant about every food and ingredient that passes our lips is unrelenting. Food fear-mongering can be found in magazines, blogs, books, and TV programming. We listen to our friends, friends of friends, and others who seem to know what they're talking about. Without even realizing it, the desire to eat healthfully can explode into uncertainty, distrust, fear, and overwhelmedness. We hear some ingredient is bad, believe it's true, and make a solemn vow to buy only fresh, unprocessed foods. Either we spend too much time trying to control everything about our eating habits or we feel overwhelmed and give up altogether. The bottom line is: Obsession with healthful eating is not healthy, and it certainly doesn't make you happy.

AM I IN FOOD JAIL?

I tend to think of foods as either "good" or "bad" based on their nutritional content.

I avoid certain foods or food groups for reasons other than an allergy or dislike of their taste or texture.

I find myself preoccupied with thoughts about food and what to eat or not eat.

I feel disappointed in myself when I "splurge" on a food I typically do not let myself eat.

I don't let myself eat "junk food" and sweets because they are not good choices.

If I eat bread or starch, it will make me gain weight.

If I eat something I shouldn't have or eat more than I wanted, I feel the need to compensate by adding exercise or planning to eat less at another time.

If I eat a fatty food, such as cheesecake or ice cream, I will gain weight.

If I eat more than my friends or family, that means I have eaten too much.

If I eat a meal or snack and I'm hungry an hour later, there's something wrong with me—I don't need that extra food.

The more you tend to agree with the above statements, the more you live by food rules and need to get out of jail!

One of my biggest grievances with food rules is how they surreptitiously steal your mental and emotional energy. These little thieves seem innocent enough, but they can keep your best asset (your brain) from more important, enjoyable work. If you find yourself caught up in moments of fear and confusion when it comes to food choices, it might be time to ask yourself: "How does this 'rule' help me create a better life?" Does it help connect you with the people you care about or help you share your gifts with the world? At best, food rules are a distraction, but most likely, they are sabotaging your best intentions to take care of yourself and enjoy your life—not just with food, but with everything you care about.

Susan was a chronic dieter who had been trying to lose weight since high school. At the suggestion of a personal trainer, she had already instituted some pretty intense food rules, eliminating some of her favorite foods, such as bread, chocolate, and french fries. Sure, Susan could follow the rules for some time, but there was always a breakdown. And when she inevitably said "screw it," she reacted by eating everything in sight, as quickly as she could manage, and then the guilt would sink in, like the weight of a thousand donuts on her conscience.

Susan felt like she would never be free from her battles with food. Over the years, she maintained a list of good and bad foods. Other people could eat the "bad" items, but she did not trust herself. It was too difficult for her to be around these foods without overdoing it. Social events were hard because she'd pay more attention to her fears and insecurities than the people at the event. Even family dinners were stressful if someone in her family offered her a food that made her feel uncomfortable.

I asked Susan if she ever considered that eliminating foods she liked made them even more irresistible. "Not really," she replied. "I just thought I was doing what I was supposed to. I don't want a life when I'm never allowed to have chocolate,

but I'm so afraid I'll overdo it, and then be all the way back where I started. That's almost worse than not having it at all."

I suggested she consider making peace with food by confronting her fears head-on and giving herself permission to eat the foods she was most afraid of. She agreed that it was worth trying a new approach. Together, we tackled her food rules one by one, giving her a new experience with the food she feared in order to rebuild her trust. For example, when she wanted to add bread back onto her menu, she would schedule it for at least one meal every day. On Monday she'd have toast with eggs and avocado, Tuesday a tuna fish sandwich, Wednesday homemade garlic bread with roasted chicken and vegetables. The fact that she was choosing to eat bread every single day gave her a reliable structure. If she had the urge to get more when it was done, she said, "Let me choose something else if I'm still hungry; I'll have more bread tomorrow." With this approach, Susan could enjoy the bread calmly, without an angry, resentful feeling.

After a few weeks of this, Susan told me, "Frankly, I lost my obsession with bread before the weekend. I knew this was going to work when it almost felt like a chore to eat my daily bread!" Legalizing bread and her other forbidden foods gave Susan the comfort and confidence that she could eat all kinds of foods in feel-good ways. She didn't panic, and usually the food she feared lost its allure when she stopped struggling so much with it.

Spiral Up
EXPRESS BODY KINDNESS WITH FOOD

Open up your journal and reflect on food choices and body kindness. What is getting in the way of expressing body kindness through what you eat? If you could gain new eating habits, what do you wish you could do effortlessly? What foods did you used to enjoy, but you've been avoiding for no good reason? Think about this: How has your attachment to food rules been harmful? How much of the good life have you missed out on when you were too preoccupied with good and bad food choices? What positive connections would you like to make to food and eating again? Think about what matters most to you. Are there helpful boundaries to guide your food choices or unhelpful, unsatisfying rules? Perhaps you think twice about noshing on a chocolate muffin in the office break room because the store-bought version just isn't as delicious as the one you can get from that bakery you love. List some actions you can take to create your new body kindness food philosophy.

How to Legalize Food

We all know it's important to eat healthful foods. However, healthful eating *patterns* are not perfect eating *rules*. Free yourself from jail and fire the "food police"—you have the keys:

BELIEVE NO FOOD IS MORALLY GOOD OR BAD. Trust your opinions about taste and enjoyment to guide your food choices. Include foods you love on your regular menu, not just for a "cheat day" or once in a blue moon.

BE SKEPTICAL OF ANY INFORMATION SENSATIONALIZING FOOD: "poison," "toxin," "never eat," or other words that trigger your fear reflexes inappropriately.

CHALLENGE YOUR OWN BELIEFS. Stop and think about why you're avoiding certain foods. Do you even remember? Is it possible what you believe may not be true?

....

GIVE YOURSELF A GET-OUT-OF-FOOD-JAIL PARTY. Make a list of foods you tend to avoid, and then serve them with other foods at a party with friends. Savor them out in the open.

....

MAKE A "FOOD FREEDOM" LIST and choose one food a week you will eat every day in a calm, pleasurable way.

....

DATE YOUR DESSERT. Come up with a special plan for enjoying a yummy cupcake that resembles how you imagine other people eat cupcakes.

Feeling absolute freedom from years of food purgatory is a journey. Try not to rush the process and be quick to forgive yourself when you slip back into old habits. **As you release yourself from moral judgments, you may find yourself noticing them everywhere you turn.** Your good friend feels guilty about something she did or didn't do. Your colleague makes a comment that suddenly makes you feel bad about the dessert you ordered with lunch. In these moments, I take a quiet deep breath, say, "Let me do me" in my head, and then completely change the subject. It also helps to recall someone I respect not giving a care about what other people think to remind myself I'm not alone.

Healthful eating is a pattern, not a rule. Trust your habits enough to be flexible. You can eat a meal on vacation, at a restaurant, or in your own home that doesn't earn a gold star, and you can enjoy the hell out of it without feeling like you should be in jail. You still remember that you love fruits and vegetables even when you don't eat them. If you're thinking, "I'm screwed. I don't trust myself at all," you're not alone. Past negative experiences can injure trust, but new positive experiences can repair it. You're not screwed. Find the courage to try to create new, positive, and joyful experiences.

....

Why I Don't Like the "Clean Eating" Label

....

I don't believe the recent "clean eating" trend that has taken over in the last few years is helpful to the majority of people, and the reasons are very simple: 1) Experts can't agree on a definition of what it actually means, and 2) "clean" implies that other eating is "dirty." The thought of uncleanliness and dirt triggers the disgust emotion. There is no reason to be disgusted by most foods. Clean eating is at best a silly fad and at worst it's a dangerous movement, fueling fear, anxiety, obsession, eating disorders, and orthorexia (an unhealthy obsession with healthful eating). It's one thing to be grateful for your food, to think about the farmer, to support a local CSA (Community Supported Agriculture), to care about where your food comes from, to aim to eat wholesome foods, but this can quickly become unhealthy and unhelpful when taken to the extreme. The only reason "clean eating" is popular is because it sells. There is no evidence to show it makes you any healthier.

How to Connect with Food Again

For many people, rebuilding a healthier relationship with food is a necessary step to truly be free from dieting, to gain confidence and feel good. Here is my three-legged stool approach to help you eat with body kindness—be hungry, balance your plate, and savor your meal.

1. Be Hungry

It probably comes as no surprise that the best time to eat is when you are hungry. It's your body's way of saying "feeeeed meeee." Recognizing hunger can be difficult for many people, and acknowledging fullness can be even more difficult. Physically, you might feel a belly growl or emptiness when you're hungry. If you eat within two hours after waking up, on most days you should experience hunger roughly every three to five hours. Hunger signals build gradually. As you digest food and have less energy available, your body begins to release hormones to increase your appetite and interest in eating.

The hungry/full system works beautifully if you work with it instead of trying to cheat it. From a body kindness perspective, any plan that tells you to fight your own biology is out of bounds. When you don't get enough food, your brain eats itself. I'm serious. It's called autophagy. Essentially it's one of the ways your body tries to compensate for the lack of food in a last-ditch effort to ward off starvation. So, if you need your brain cells like I do, then eating enough food is key. You will feel a serious energy decline and loss of focus and concentration if you don't eat enough. And we all know someone who has "hanger issues," right? It's funny to joke about it, but mood fluctuations are a legitimate hormonal response when your body and brain don't get the fuel they need to function adequately.

QUICK SNACKS TO
AVOID GETTING "HANGRY"

FRUIT such as apples, bananas, kiwifruit, dried plums, and dates on their own or with peanut, almond, cashew, or sunflower butter.

DIP IT! Blend plain yogurt with 2 tablespoons of peanut butter or fresh herbs for a dip with your favorite fruits and vegetables.

CHEESE WITH VEGETABLES OR FRUIT such as cucumbers, peppers, celery, carrots, tomatoes, kiwifruit, grapes, mandarin orange slices, red grapefruit, and pears.

HARD-BOILED EGG WITH AVOCADO. Take a whole egg and place it in the pit of half an avocado. Top with a bit of salt and pepper or hot sauce.

TUNA WITH AVOCADO. Fill the pit of half an avocado with tuna (I love tuna packed in olive oil). Top with a squeeze of lemon.

HUMMUS WITH PITA AND VEGETABLES. Cut half a whole-wheat pita into triangles and use veggies as dippers with store-bought hummus.

DIY TRAIL MIX. Combine your favorite nuts such as pistachios, peanuts, and almonds, dried fruit (plums, mangoes, raisins, cranberries), chocolate chips, and dry cereal.

TIP: Get help from the grocery store. Many retailers provide grab-and-go snacks like cheese, guacamole, nuts, precut vegetables and fruits, KIND bars, fruit leather, single-serve chips, and more. If you can't find ready-to-go snacks, make your own ahead of time to make "hangry" history.

2. Balance Your Plate

One way to increase the variety of foods you eat and simplify decision-making is by using the balanced plate method to guide your food choices. The perk is that there is no need to restrict or measure your food and no calorie counting or scrutinizing of ingredients. All you need is a pair of eyes and an elementary understanding of fractions. The concept is so simple it almost feels like it can't possibly work, but it does. (And just think of all the free time you'll have when you aren't entering every morsel of food into a calorie counting app!)

When you look at the balanced plates, you may notice one important feature: Within the realm of your preferences, plants should be the basis of your food intake. Why? They offer fiber, vitamins, and minerals for nourishment. One-half to three quarters of the plate diagrams are plant foods—fruits,

HELP WITH HUNGER
HOW FULL IS YOUR TANK?

Think of your stomach like a gas tank signaling hunger & fullness.

TYPICAL HUNGER
You have some fuel but need more to keep your energy going. Plan on eating soon—make sure you have food and time to focus on eating.

1/4

RUNNING ON FUMES
aka "hangry."
You probably waited too long. Eat now, but relax; take your time. Try to avoid getting here in future.

EMPTY

CONTENTED
You don't feel the need to eat right now, and you're not really thinking about it. You might feel this way between meals. You're more focused on things like work or fun.

JUST RIGHT
The "feel good" place to stop when you're eating. You may have room for more, but it would probably overfill you. Remember the time it takes for the fullness message to reach your brain—up to 30 minutes.

½

¾

UH OH, TOO FULL
It's an uncomfortable feeling that you exceeded your limit. Try to avoid.

FULL

vegetables, beans, legumes, seeds, nuts, and whole-grain foods. Plant-based eating is in line with the USDA's *Dietary Guidelines for Americans*, which is updated every five years by a panel of nutrition scientists. As long as you work on adequately filling this part of the plate MOST of the time, the rest of your decisions become less important (and less difficult).

Don't forget to save room for my favorite part of the balanced plate approach: It's called eating whatever the heck you want. (You rebel, you!) I'm talking some meals that have no vegetables or fruits at all. Life is meant to be lived fully—not monitored and morseled out into perfect portions. But what about health? Enjoying pizza, french fries, and hot fudge sundaes does not *give* someone diabetes. But it might just give them joy once in a while. We've all heard of someone's Aunty Betty who lived to be 101 eating bacon and mayonnaise sandwiches every day from her easy chair. And we all know people who seem to have done everything by the book yet still struggle with unexplainable health challenges. While your lifestyle choices can impact health, so can genetics, the environment, and even socioeconomic status. I want to enjoy the years I have on this planet, and taking pleasure in flexible, adventurous eating fits my definition of "the good life" more than forcing myself to always adhere to a balanced plate—or else!

Ways the Balanced Plate Works for You

SUPPORTS YOUR DAY-TO-DAY ENERGY. When you eat better, you tend to feel better, sleep better, and as a collective result, have more energy.

MAXIMIZES YOUR DIGESTIVE HEALTH. Foods rich in fiber will keep your digestive system running smoothly, helping you absorb nutrients, which then fuel all your other body functions.

STRENGTHENS YOUR GUT MICRO-BIOME. One hundred trillion of your body's best friends, otherwise known as the bacteria living in your gut, make up what is known as your microbiome—considered your "second brain." It's key to regulating your mood through the signaling of neurotransmitters and production of serotonin, which I like to think of as the "keep calm and carry on" hormone. When you eat certain foods, like bananas, artichokes, and kiwi, you get undigestable fibers called prebiotics that feed your "good bacteria." Eating fermented foods like yogurt, kefir, kimchi, and miso gives you a direct dose of probiotics to help populate your gut. You can also take probiotic supplements. All these efforts will help the most beneficial bacteria thrive in your gut and keep potentially harmful viruses and bacteria from taking up residence.

Spiral Up
BUILD BALANCED PLATES
EAT WELL WITHOUT OVERTHINKING IT

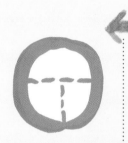

THE STANDARD GUIDE FOR AN IDEALLY BALANCED PLATE.

Half fruits and vegetables, one quarter whole grains, one quarter protein-rich foods.

Use it when you feel your normal level of hunger.

This is a good guide for meal planning and grocery shopping.

THIS VERSION BOOSTS PROTEIN AND STARCH.

One third each fruits and vegetables, whole grains, and protein-rich foods.

If you're hungrier than normal or dining out, this plate may fit better.

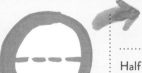

THIS PLATE STILL PLACES A PRIORITY ON FRUITS AND VEGGIES.

Half fruits and vegetables and half whole grains, protein, or a combination of the two.

It also acknowledges that sometimes you want a big hunk o' protein or a comforting portion of pasta.

BOOSTS YOUR IMMUNITY. Your immune system is constantly fighting any potentially harmful pathogens that make it into your body. Eating foods with the antioxidants vitamins A, C, and E help keep your immune system strong. The yellow-flesh SunGold kiwifruit has three times the vitamin C of oranges. Also try blueberries, grapefruit, broccoli, avocado, mangoes, carrots, sweet potatoes, seeds, and nuts.

HELPS YOUR BODY NATURALLY DETOX-IFY. You don't need cleanses or detoxes because your liver and kidneys do all the hard work for you. Your liver sifts through every ounce of blood looking for anything it does not like and getting rid of it (like alcohol, prescription drugs, or other body toxins). Then your kidneys help turn it into waste so when you "go" it goes bye-bye. Keep this process operating smoothly by drinking plenty of water and keeping alcohol intake in check.

FIGHTS INFLAMMATION. Sometimes your body responds to injury or illness with pain and discomfort in an attempt to heal itself—this can also happen with food intolerance or sensitivities or certain chronic illnesses such as Crohn's disease, lupus, or arthritis. The majority of leafy greens, fruits, and other healthful foods like nuts, olive oil, celery, beets, salmon, tuna, and anchovies are anti-inflammatory. This can help decrease generalized inflammation in your body.

People who are flexible with their choices have more self-control in the long run. It might sound counterintuitive, but giving yourself some rewarding pleasure now (with reasonable self-control) can actually help you avoid self-sabotage later on. Instead of completely avoiding Grandma's delicious mac-n-cheese recipe, it's much more realistic to enjoy a satisfying portion as part of a well-rounded meal. If this sounds like it requires superhuman power, consider how taking the time to slowly savor your meal and get comfortably full can be satisfying and help prevent mindless eating later on.

It's OK if following the balanced plate is a challenge. Start where you are, working with your preferences, and try to be flexible and creative with meal planning. Many of my clients want to know how they can "healthify" their favorite meals, so I've compiled a few of my favorite ways to turn an old classic into a more balanced plate.

3. Savor Your Meal

Savor means to taste food and enjoy it completely—something we rarely do anymore because who has the time? Making an effort to savor your meal is part of the body kindness plan because savoring is all about connection and pleasure. What we eat impacts our mind and spirit just as much as our bodies. When you engage in food savoring behaviors, you're bound to spiral up. My plan to help you savor your food more involves mindfulness—emphasizing enhancements to flavor when you prepare the meal and mindful eating practices to help you enjoy it more fully. Both these factors will help you self-regulate how much food you eat. (You don't need a diet to tell you that anymore! Hooray!)

Somewhere along the way, butter and salt ended up on the same blacklist as potato chips, and in their place landed a steaming bowl of plain broccoli. Butter and salt are among the top flavor enhancers, so I encourage you

Spiral Up
HOW TO HEALTHIFY

* **Pasta:** Try pasta noodles made from pulses (a collective term for beans and legumes—like lentils and chickpeas), use whole-wheat pasta, or substitute anywhere from half to all of your pasta noodles with noodles you make from zucchini or squash using an inexpensive kitchen tool called a spiralizer.

Boost your helping of veggies in the sauce. Starting with canned, crushed tomatoes, add mushrooms (pulsed in a food processor to the size of ground beef), plus any other vegetable (cooked or raw) you have on hand. Don't like chunky? You can toss your sauce in a blender for a smooth consistency. Make a pesto sauce with broccoli, spinach, kale, cauliflower, or a combination.

* **Burgers:** Blend half the ground beef with sautéed mushrooms from the food processor. Nobody will ask "where's the beef?" and the mushrooms add flavor. It's practically a salad!

* **Mac-n-cheese:** The cheese is the star here. Rather than try to cut it back, add a vegetable puree that blends right in. Pureed cauliflower and butternut squash are my favorites. Serve up with a side of broccoli. (Kid-Tested Meal Plan: mac-n-cheese with "little trees"!) It works with the boxed stuff, too.

to put them back on the table if it will help increase vegetable consumption. A little goes a long way. Exploring new and interesting flavors, such as salty and sweet combinations, can make eating well more exciting too.

Take a Break to Enjoy What You Eat

In America, we don't make space for uninterrupted, joyful eating like other cultures do. We dash down the hall with a kale smoothie in our hand. No time to chew! Giving yourself room to eat without distractions can make all the difference in how you experience the taste of food and, ultimately, your satisfaction. The most logical place to eat is at a table, but anywhere you feel calm and focused on the process of eating and can connect to your body's cues is a good place to eat. A park bench on a sunny day is often more desirable than eating at your desk while answering a few more emails. Listening to music is more enjoyable and less distracting than watching television. Standing in front of the refrigerator or sitting behind the steering wheel—these are not the best places to eat and maintain focus and satisfaction.

Mindful eating involves choosing to sit down in a comfortable space to eat (not on the sofa) and removing distractions, like your TV and computer, to enjoy the experience of eating. When eating mindfully, you focus on appreciating that moment, whether you're eating the most amazing food of your life or making your way through "meh" leftovers. Mindful eaters are less likely to overeat and more likely to feel good about their choices. Initially, it may be an effort to make time for eating, but the truth is you can eat mindfully whether it's one minute or sixty minutes. And once you integrate this practice into your daily routine you'll wonder why on earth you ever thought eating in the car was a reasonable way to consume food!

Become an Intuitive Eater

There is no right or wrong way to eat when you let your body's natural wisdom guide you. This includes your ability to perceive when you are hungry and need nourishment, noticing when you are getting full, recognizing when you are satisfied as an indicator that you're getting enough to eat, and using your wisdom to choose when it's the right time to acknowledge a craving and when it's not. We are born knowing these things. When babies are hungry, they cry. When they are satisfied, they relax, sleep, or smile. Unfortunately, our entire culture (and sometimes even our loving parents) participates in separating us from this innate wisdom. For the most part, eating should feel good before, during, and afterward.

Most women I meet feel disconnected from their bodies and these biological cues. If you've dieted, cleansed, or restricted your food in the past, if you eat emotionally and sometimes overeat, you may be able to relate to this disconnection. It's not easy to make food choices when you're trying to control your biological need for nourishment. Intuitive eating may be an approach for you. I practice intuitive eating, and this is my favorite method to use with clients who want help making food choices that don't involve fads, diets, and rules.

The Intuitive Eating Model

Intuitive eating is a form of attunement of mind, body, and food. It's a model developed by Evelyn Tribole and Elyse Resch, coauthors of the book *Intuitive Eating*, with three key elements: 1) Eat for physical rather than emotional reasons, 2) rely on internal hunger and satiety cues, and 3) give yourself unconditional permission to eat. This includes permission to eat what you want, as much as you want, and weigh what you will, rather than trying to control your weight. (This is the part where I usually expect clients to look for the nearest escape route from my office!) For some people, the mere thought of eating "whatever" unleashes a fear of uncontrollable behaviors and weight gain. But that's all it is: fear, deeply buried under years of struggle and frustration.

The intuitive eating model is positive, free of food rules and diets, and it promotes a self-respecting approach to eating, where hunger drives the decision to eat and fullness drives the decision to stop. During the process of eating, it's important to be "tuned in" to food and eating, with a keen sense of awareness.

If you're thinking that this sounds like mindfulness or mindful eating, you're right (sort of). Both mindful eating and intuitive eating can help facilitate normal eating. Intuitive eating is a broader philosophy that incorporates mindfulness, as well as principles like rejecting the diet mentality and engaging in physical activity for the sake of feeling good. Perhaps most significantly, intuitive eating has been validated by many research studies as a healthful practice. People who eat intuitively are more likely to improve their eating habits, lifestyle, and body image. They are less likely to be depressed, anxious, and have low self-esteem. **Over thirty studies show that people who practice intuitive eating instead of dieting**

CHOOSE MINDFUL EATING

ENJOY EATING WITH ALL YOUR SENSES

You'll notice new tastes and textures in even the most familiar food when you eat mindfully.

Slowing down before you start eating helps you establish a calmer pace of eating.

You'll feel good about your food choices when you seek pleasurable eating experiences.

As you eat mindfully, you'll notice fullness and avoid overeating.

How Much Time Do You Have?

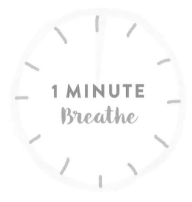

1 MINUTE
Breathe

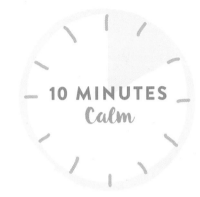

10 MINUTES
Calm

TAKE FIVE DEEP breaths before your first bite. With each breath, think of a different person you'd like to send some love and happiness to. You'll start the meal more relaxed and be able to eat and digest better.

AFTER YOUR "BREATHING BREAK" take that first bite of food. Really pay attention. Chew it as if you were discovering it for the first time. Take your time with each bite for the first 10 minutes of the meal.

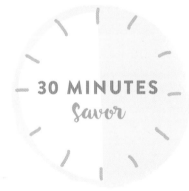

30 MINUTES
Savor

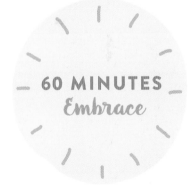

60 MINUTES
Embrace

EXPERIENCE YOUR ENTIRE meal mindfully. Notice everything your meal has to offer using your sight, senses of smell and taste, and physical sensation. Notice what you're thinking and feeling and whether any memories arise.

PREPARE YOUR MEAL mindfully. No matter how easy your recipe is to prepare you will gain so much more by slowing down. Notice the sounds, smells, aromas, and physicality of preparing your meal.

improve their heart health (measured blood pressure, blood lipids, and cardiorespiratory fitness) even in the absence of weight loss. My three-legged stool approach for making food choices is inspired by the intuitive eating model.

Choosing to Eat with Body Kindness

When I think of eating with body kindness, it brings to mind a feeling of openness in my heart and mind. I feel interest, wonder, and excitement about the food that is in front of me, and an upward spiral of happiness takes over, especially if it's as delicious as I hoped.

Imagine being adventurous and curious about the taste of a new dessert without saying, "I'll need to make up for this tomorrow!" Keep in mind, being flexible does not mean you don't give a crap about what you put into your body. It means you understand that food is only part of healthful living and you trust that there's room for give-and-take. When you say good-bye to food rules, you say hello to freedom and peace. Feeling guilty for eating is like feeling guilty for being happy or punishing yourself for having an afternoon of fun with a friend.

Body kindness food choices are personal decisions, and they aren't up for judgment or unsolicited advice. Listen to your heart and body and then embrace your preferences unapologetically. Give up the "virtue" of all choices and start thinking about the choices you *really* want to make. Eat cake if you want cake and kale if you want kale, but don't make it about anything more than it really is: just one of the many millions of food choices you are going to make in your lifetime. You'll enjoy the cake and the kale much more when they aren't tied to your worthiness.

BODY KINDNESS REFLECTION: Journal for fifteen minutes about food choices. How do you express body kindness with food, and how would you like to improve? What steps could you take to live more peacefully and healthfully with your food choices?

"People who love to eat are always the best people."

—Julia Child

Chapter 3

Fitness for *Your* Life

Choose What Works for You

Philosophy

Fitness is a measurement of several factors, including heart and muscle strength and joint flexibility. Much like how you take your coffee, fitness routines are a matter of personal preference. If you want to form new exercise habits, choose activities that are meaningful to you and workable in your life. Your amazing body was born to move, and your body kindness practice should include a sustainable exercise "sweet spot" where enjoyment, consistency, and health converge. Start simple, like a six-year-old who just loves to move, and it's more likely you'll learn to enjoy fitness for life—that is the body kindness imperative. Keep moving, every chance you get—because you want to take care of yourself.

BODY KINDNESS PILLARS
Feel Body Kindness in Movement

LOVE: Choose exercises that bring you pleasure and joy, and trust that whatever you decide, it's enough because it fits your preferences.

CONNECT: Listen to your body for signals, such as "increase intensity," "slow down," "take a break."

CARE: Make some amount of feel-good movement a daily priority because your body needs it and you want to care for your body.

We Are Made to Move

From the time we are babies learning what our bodies can do, to the rambunctious, full-bodied movement of childhood, we are born to move. But then we are asked to sit on our pockets in kindergarten circle time, and from there life gradually becomes less about moving and more about strengthening our ability to sit still. Between business meetings, lunch with friends, and family dinners followed by evenings on our comfy sofa—not to mention the convenience of modern transportation—our daily rituals are built around immobility. And because we're not walking miles in search of food or plowing the field all day for exercise, this means we have to actively seek out the movements and activities our bodies were meant to be engaged in.

The most important decision you can make about exercise is simply to move your body more often with joy and satisfaction. My goal for this chapter is to help you say "Yes!" to fitness by addressing common barriers, sharing ideas for activities you can do anywhere, and encouraging you to challenge yourself. The body kindness mindset means saying good-bye to punishing and compensatory exercise routines to make way for a whole new approach to fitness. If exercise is not something you do regularly, I'll help you create a dream routine and turn your thoughts from "I should work out" to "I can't miss my workout."

Spiral Up

Think about being six years old. Remember the hopscotch jump? Feet apart, jump forward on one foot, feet apart. Remember jumping rope, riding your bike, and playing tag? When you were younger, moving was second nature. If you tried one of these right now, just the action alone may give you a little youthful joy. Reflect on how satisfied you are with your current physical activity. Would you like it to be more playful, interesting, or fun? Even though a lot has changed since your Hula-Hooping days, it's never too late to choose fitness for life.

All you need for an ideal fitness plan are two simple things: 1) any activity you're willing to do that gets your heart rate going and 2) a commitment to start. That's it.

The simpler you make your plan, the more likely you are to succeed. Take a few minutes and write a fitness reflection in your body kindness journal. Do you consider fitness a mandatory form of self-care? Why or why not? How satisfied are you with your exercise habits? What would you change if you could? When I say "exercise" you think _____. How do you feel when you move your body, both positive and negative? What are the reasons you give for not doing a workout? What would make choosing fitness over other ways of spending time easier for you? Think about what would need to change in your life to make room for exercising your way.

Motivation, Wherefore Art Thou?

You water your plants, you feed your cat, and you move your butt. Exercise is just one of those non-negotiable to-dos on the checklist of life. Unlike eating and drinking, we can skip exercise for quite a long time without too many bodily complaints, and the downsides of inactivity are often tolerable enough to ignore. There's no looming crisis forcing it to happen every day, and there are plenty of other things we could do, should do, and would rather do. I've learned from my clients that in order to "Just say yes" to movement instead of "Yes, but . . ." each person has to find her own three *W*'s—Why, What, and When.

WHY: *Why* you want to exercise uncovers personally meaningful benefits to help you take exercise from a "should do" to a "will do."

WHAT: *What* do you enjoy doing? Find a rewarding and interesting activity.

WHEN: *When* will you do it? Having a set schedule turns the desire to exercise into an actionable plan.

Your Appearance Is Not Your "Why"

A popular reason people give for working out is because they want to look good, whether they are trying to lose weight, tone up, or maintain their present physique. While I could list dozens of proven benefits of exercise (we all know them), vanity doesn't rise to the top. But I get it.

If our social media news feeds and the latest infomercials were any indicator, you would think we're all motivated by sweaty bodies with photoshopped arms, impossible waistlines, and abs that "pop for days." This type of "fitspiration" places value on appearance over health. But the ugly truth is that many fitness images you see are not necessarily those of healthy people. They are fitness models, fitness gurus (or aspiring gurus), and regular people obsessed with how they look, not how healthy they are. Sure, maybe a few are genetic anomalies, like 0.0001 percent of the population. Still, they should not be the image of the fitness standard we're all striving to attain.

You don't create a genuine, lifelong love of fitness by forcing yourself to go to uncomfortable exercise extremes or demanding that your body take on an unnatural appearance. Sustainable health and fitness, the kind that nourishes your body and your soul, can come only from committing to a flexible way of moving that you find satisfying and enjoyable.

Breaking news: You can be fit *and* fat. Inactivity, not fatness, is linked to mortality and heart disease. A fat, *fit* person has half the risk of death of an *unfit* person at the same weight. Whatever measure you are using for health—the scale, the calorie counter on the elliptical machine, or your fitness tracker—these devices don't show you reductions in blood pressure, blood sugar, blood lipids, or stress levels, or improvements in mood. I call the famously unhelpful body mass index (BMI) the "BS Measurement of Inaccuracy." This torture tool is nothing more than a simple math equation created in 1832 to label the "normal man," and medical researchers started using it in the 1970s as a cheap, universal way to estimate relative body fat across populations, not individuals.

Today's BMI calculators are based on height and weight measurements of adult white males, and don't account for gender, genetics, muscle mass, activity, or diverse populations. My professional advice is to run far and fast from anyone trying to use BMI as an indicator of your health status.

Research has continually proven that the fitness industry's focus on physical appearance does very little to actually get people up and moving. In fact, this kind of guilt-based pseudo-motivation hinders many people from making a long-term commitment to exercise, and actually harms body image. Why? Because when appearance is the primary goal, there will always be work to do and you will never be satisfied, even when your behavior and your physical health indicate you're doing well. When you fall short of perfection (not looking like the instructor or the person next to you, not losing the weight you hoped for), it feels like a failure and your motivation falls by the wayside. Thankfully, there is a growing movement of fitness professionals who are fighting back against the notion that exercise should be grounded in achieving a better appearance. So if you're considering hiring someone to help you reach your fitness goals, I encourage you to seek out experts who focus on self-care and inner strength vs. pounds lost and lifted. They should be just as interested in how you feel as in how many reps you can do. Fitness is a commitment to caring for both mind and body. Make sure the fitness experts you hire share your philosophy and understand your boundaries. If they aren't enhancing your experience, let them know what you need or find someone else who can help. Respectful care for enjoyable exercise routines is not "nice to have"; it's essential for body kindness.

Sometimes I get the feeling that people think I don't care about appearance at all—as if I don't believe in showers or makeup. I love showers and I love looking and feeling my best. I also like the idea of being "in shape"—*my shape*. I see myself as a fit person because of everything I do for fitness. I love how being fit helps me fully engage in life—like having the stamina to do housework (which can double as exercise, by the way) and the endurance to play with my energetic daughters. Looking at my arms, you might not be able to tell that yesterday I held a headstand pose for five minutes without the wall for support, but I still felt a wonderful sense of accomplishment. And my thighs don't say, "Look everyone! This amazing woman ran five miles today!" My body does tell a story, but it's not necessarily one that can be measured by eyeballs. I intentionally choose different ways to measure health and fitness because I don't ever want my appearance to dictate my success or undercut my achievements. This is the wish I have for you too.

A Body Kindness Movement Manifesto

I RESPECT MY BODY AND MOVE MY BODY EVERY DAY as an intentional demonstration of love and respect for myself.

MY MOVEMENT IS FOCUSED ON THE PRESENT MOMENT, without comparison to past performance, other people, or anything that takes my thoughts away from appreciating what my body can do.

WHEN I'M ACTIVE, I SEEK OUT MEANINGFUL, IMMEDIATE REWARDS in how I feel and how much energy I have to do things I care about.

I MIGHT NOT ALWAYS FEEL IN THE MOOD TO EXERCISE, but I can always commit to some movement that's satisfying and good enough.

MY MOVEMENT IS A JUDGMENT-FREE ZONE. There are no good or bad, right or wrong activities. My enjoyment counts more than my calorie burn.

MY BODY IS NOT FAILING ME IF SOMETHING IS DIFFICULT. Challenges are an opportunity to grow my strengths and learn something new.

I CALL THE SHOTS, and if things don't feel right, I can make an adjustment. If I notice pain, I stop and investigate the cause.

MY STRONGEST MUSCLE IS MY OPEN HEART that holds me with kindness no matter what.

WHAT'S YOUR *WHY*?

This manifesto suggests a flexible approach to fitness, where your happiness and well-being come first. When you embrace movement as a way of life, common barriers begin to melt away. Just like other areas of body kindness, the most important way to make a lifelong commitment to fitness is to focus on your *Why*. Once you've identified why exercise is important to you, then you can move on to the next two *W*'s: the *What* and the *When*. You can also continue using the DARN exercise from Chapter 1 (see page 36) to help you visualize the actions that will help you reach your fitness goals. Imagine yourself ten or fifteen years from now. What do you want to be able to enjoy in life, and what small changes can you make to see that through? By integrating these future-oriented thoughts into your fitness plan, you are providing internal motivation to help you reach your goals.

I used to exercise to try to fit myself into some version of perfection that I hoped to see in the mirror—my idea of what a successful registered dietitian should look like in order to be worthy of a full roster of clients and a busy schedule. These days, the motivation behind my workouts is having the energy I need and honoring my commitment to sacred "me time" for movement. Consider how you might translate a fitness to-do list into a fitness *Why* statement. Even if you proudly exercise regularly and wouldn't

Spiral Up
MOVEMENT MOTIVATIONS

Choose one or more of the statements from the body kindness movement manifesto on page 72 that really resonate with you, or create your own positive, inspiring messages about movement. Put them on sticky notes or make pretty index cards and place them somewhere you know you'll see them when you need a boost of encouragement. Here are a few ideas from clients about where and how they've used *movement motivations* to strengthen their fitness goals:

★ "*On the mirror in my bathroom* because this is where I feel most vulnerable, seeing all the flaws of my naked body, and I need a gentle reminder of all I do to take care of myself."

★ "*My workout room* so I'm reminded that it's not how much I do, but that I'm doing it, and that if I'm not having fun I should change things up."

★ "*In my journal.* I use it as my bookmark and read it before each new entry."

★ "*Next to the remote control.* When I think about turning on the TV, it reminds me to think about my choices. I can always do a few squats before I sit down or during commercials if I haven't exercised yet. Sometimes I'll skip the TV and do a workout first, then reward myself with a little uninterrupted TV time later."

★ "*On my monitor at work and in my home office* to give me the kick in the butt to at least stand up and do a few calf lifts or simple stretches while I'm staring at the screen."

dream of missing it, it's worth asking "Why?" Your motivation should be positive, encouraging, and body loving (or at least body appreciating). The ultimate goal is to shift your inner dialogue (more on this later) away from exercising just to prevent fatness, to earn the right to eat dessert, or wear a crop top. You are more likely to form a solid connection with your body and develop a lifelong habit when you make movement meaningful and fun!

Why Isn't Everyone on the Exercise Drug?

Unlike dieting, there are virtually no downsides to regular, enjoyable exercise. Being active makes you a healthier, stronger, and happier person. If you've ever felt clearheaded and calm after a workout, you've experienced the drug-free way to regulate your mood through physical activity. In some studies, exercise has been shown to be as effective as Prozac in treating depression. Exercise also improves outcomes in the treatment of cancer, heart disease, diabetes, and nearly every chronic condition. People who exercise regularly are more creative, more productive, and more resilient in times of stress.

In spite of all these benefits, the average American moves less than twenty minutes a day, and one third of adults report exercising only once a week or not at all. If we're going to escape this trap and choose a life of true fitness, we need to focus on our *Why*, and then on the immediate, tangible benefits that come from exercise.

Feeling tired and groggy in the afternoon? Stop daydreaming about a nap or coffee and go for a walk. When you're tired, exercise may seem like the last logical thing you should do. But post-exercise energy bursts are natural outcomes of your physiology. Moving your body recruits your heart and lungs to work together to pump blood faster, bringing more nutrients to every part of your body, strengthening every cell, and allowing your muscles to utilize available energy. With exercise, your muscles intentionally develop tiny tears and then rebuild them with new fibers, making you stronger for the next bout of activity. The more fit you are, the more energy-creating potential you have. Fit people have more mitochondria—tiny powerhouses inside the cells whose job it is to turn glucose (i.e., sugar) into energy with every muscle contraction.

Spiral Up

INSTANT GRATIFICATION

Here are my personal top five body kindness motivation mindsets that capitalize on the instant benefits of exercise.

* **I need a break.** When my productivity takes a nosedive, I power up with exercise and reboot my mental computer.

* **I need a pick-me-up.** When I'm feeling negative emotions, movement is a natural mood booster.

* **It's more fun than work.** When I'm struggling through any work problem, I inevitably feel like a pile of poo at some point. Movement is my form of productive procrastination and usually makes me more optimistic about the tasks ahead.

* **It's my chance to connect.** Whether with a friend or myself, exercise is my momentary escape and bond-building time.

* **Because I can.** When I'm dragging my feet, I remember that I have feet and legs and a glorious body that craves movement. Out of love for myself and gratitude for my health, I choose to move.

When you finish a workout, your body is flooded with nutrient-rich blood and endorphins. It's like waking your body up from the inside. The energy yield from movement sets you on an upward spiral path. You can reduce fatigue by as much as 65 percent by participating in regular, low-intensity exercise like walking. Instead of just surviving the day (which can feel like a pretty admirable goal in and of itself sometimes), a commitment to more movement will make each day more productive and meaningful.

Exercise Heals Body Image

Not surprisingly, people who have negative feelings about their weight or shape are less likely to exercise (especially as a form of self-care), but scientific literature indicates that those with the poorest body image receive the richest psychological benefits from exercise. You might think body image improves as a result of weight loss or changes in body composition, but that's not what the data shows. At best, actual measurable improvements in fitness (such as pounds and inches lost) play a minor role in creating a positive body image. The greatest improvements in body image come from believing that exercise is meaningful. When a person chooses to focus on why exercise matters, and when they acknowledge their efforts instead of their appearance, they have a healthier body image. Self-efficacy also has a direct and powerful impact. By engaging in enjoyable and interesting physical activity, a person's belief in their capabilities naturally improves. They begin to change how they see themselves and develop a new exercise mindset that fuels lasting habits.

Show Me the Money: Investing in the Bank of You

"If I gave you a million dollars, would you invest it or would you squander it?" That's how Coach Dave Egnatuk started every physical fitness class he taught at Albion College. I remember daydreaming about all the things I could get for a million bucks when he first asked our Healthy Living class this question. I wanted a private island in the Caribbean (too bad $1 million wasn't nearly enough!). As tempting as our dreams of frivolous spending were, Coach Egnatuk still managed to take hold and convince a bunch of eighteen-year-olds that we were already wealthy in terms of our health. "The human body is worth over a million dollars if you add up the potential value of all your parts, and the daily choices you make are about whether you choose to invest or squander what you've been given." Then he went on to acknowledge all the crazy things typical college kids do (lots of squandering). "But you don't have to sacrifice your health. You can choose to invest in health."

Coach Egnatuk shared a powerful story illustrating how our commitment to physical activity might one day save our lives. One of his former students had a sudden heart attack at age twenty-three. Because he was physically active, however, his body had developed extra circulation around his heart, a common adaptation that can occur in active people. It served as a natural bypass from the larger blocked blood vessels. That young man survived, giving credit to his superior physical health. He went on to have a family, start a company, and build a good life for himself.

One of Coach Egnatuk's favorite sayings was "It's a great day to be alive! You're young and physically fit. Let's get to work!" I credit him with teaching me that investing in health was my decision, an opportunity that presented itself every day. I didn't realize it at the time, but Coach Egnatuk was teaching me optimism—arguably one of the most important character traits in one's life. To this day, recalling his inspiring declarations reminds me that I have many gifts to appreciate—my life and my health are tops on that list. And no matter how hard he challenged us, I always felt better after his class (thank you, endorphins). How can you use physical activities to invest in yourself the body kindness way?

Taking Action: What and When

Once you figure out your personal motivation, my next advice for anyone trying to start a new fitness routine (or revitalize an old one) is to begin planning and doing as soon as possible, in whatever small way you can. There will be challenges and roadblocks along the way (don't worry, I've got plans to help you get around those), but the sooner you set one foot in front of the other (literally) the sooner you get to experience the upward spirals of energy that will help you start running toward your *Why*.

I've been committed to fitness longer than I've been married, but my *Why*, *What*, and *When* have all changed over the years. I can honestly say that my current exercise goals come from a place of body loving. But it wasn't always this way. My relationship with fitness was born out of experimentation, experience, and changing desires. When I became a certified aerobics instructor at eighteen years old, I was the one saying "It's bikini season, laaaaaddddiiiiessss . . . four more pulses!" (Shaking my head at my younger, less wise self.) But that's what's messed up about our culture. We have to fight the urge to equate fitness with body changes because it's been drilled into us. Work through whatever "stuff" you have to in order to get to a better place with fitness. I encourage you to keep an open mind until the time comes when you can confidently say you've found your personal fitness "fit."

What you do is up to you. Many of my clients find a renewed energy for fitness when they try new activities. Consider choosing three new things you've been curious about doing. Over time your body adapts to the same old same old and you get bored—even if it's something you love. You may need a new experience or a different twist. Clients have bounced into the room saying, "I tried Aqua Zumba and it was so much fun!" If you love yoga, check out a different studio or try aerial yoga for an entirely new experience. You might consider changing up the places you normally go for a walk (try the beach, the woods, a trail, the fancy neighborhood next to yours). If you enjoyed sports in high school, or think you'd like sports activities over gym workouts, then go in that direction. If you decide to stretch your comfort zone, plan on that first-day-of-school awkwardness, but commit ahead of time to going anyway. You will never know what it's really like until you get in there and try it for yourself.

Roadblocks and Detours on Your Fitness Journey

O ne of the top frustrations I hear from clients is "I *know* I need to exercise, Rebecca. I *want* to exercise. But why is it so hard to make it happen sometimes?" We all deal with the temptation of blowing off workouts. Use the reasons why you exercise or want to get started as a quick reality check for decision-making.

I've identified five of the most common mental challenges we face when it comes to exercise, along with my best techniques for navigating around them. These can happen to anyone at any time but especially to people who are trying to establish or re-establish workout routines.

Roadblock #1: No Time

"I'm too busy." "I work full-time." "I have young children." This category often includes both the overworked business executive and the stay-at-home parent.

No matter how you phrase it, lack of time is the most popular reason we all have for skipping a workout. But I'm ready to call everybody's bluff on that one—and I'll let you take a wild guess what too many of us are spending our time on. Exactly—Netflix, Facebook, and the like. If you had to choose between building movement into every aspect of your day or sitting all day and working out for a half hour three times a week, I'd vote for more daily movement. You can burn energy doing leisurely things you love and crossing errands off your to-do list. Just do them in the most active way possible. So take a fresh look at how you spend your time, and list as many ideas as you can find for fitness. The more repetitive you can be, the fewer decisions you'll have to make; you just do it. Walk or bike your work commute, walk to pick up lunch, walk during a lunch break, run as many errands on foot before or after work as you can. At home, turn housework into a workout. Take a quick jog up the stairs as often as you can, instead of leaving your junk on the bottom stair piling up! You can do activities even in the most minute pockets of time. It's your habit of saying "I can't" that's getting in your way of even starting.

Luckily there are still clear health benefits from short, intense interval workouts, and plenty of low-tech, no-tech, and hi-tech ways to make it happen. Look up HIIT or MIIT (high- or moderate-intensity interval training) and you'll find a plethora of routines you can do in any amount of time. Check out the Johnson & Johnson Official 7 Minute Workout app, and squeeze in a quick session while you wait for pasta to boil or for the kids to get in the car! It provides movement instructions, a timer, and visual cues for easy use during workouts. I like to use this app on days I can't make it to yoga or my solid-core class, exercises I love, but that take the better part of an hour. You can even get more out of simple bodyweight movements using a Tabata timer. A Tabata is a timed period of work followed by a period of rest, repeated as many times as you want. Set the timer, and it will do the thinking for you. Tabata Timer is one free app. Choose just one or two of the movements listed. You can get a workout in as little as four minutes, or do multiple Tabatas for more volume. I also love *The Burst! Workout*—a book full of ten-minute circuit exercises you can do anytime, anywhere. Look online, ask for recommendations, and keep searching for fitness routines that fit your needs.

Roadblock #2: "I'm just too overwhelmed!"

Even if you have plenty of exercise ideas, you might still put it off because of competing priorities—work, home, family, friends. You suffer from action paralysis because you have grandiose ideas of what exercise needs to be in order to be good enough. **The best exercise is the one you finish. That's it. Saying *not right now* over and over is as good as saying *never*.** Your brain cannot create a habit without first doing the activity you want it to learn. It's not enough to intend to exercise, and then skip it nine times out of ten. Making fitness a body kindness choice means that sometimes you'll send in store-bought cupcakes just so you can make it to yoga class, or you'll just get up from your computer and walk out the door because you need to get on with your life. Most days we don't finish what we want. If you're genuinely struggling with an overbooked calendar, consider which of your commitments you can shift to include exercise. Instead of meeting a friend for happy hour, ask her to make it a walk-and-talk, followed up with a nice sparkling water or herbal tea. Those who sweat together, stay together! Embrace the fitness ideas from the "no time" roadblock on page 78 and make movement one of your top priorities.

Roadblock #3: It's Not Fun

If you are excited about your exercise activities, you are more likely to get started and will procrastinate less often. Make it more fun (or at least less dreadful) with music, a great audiobook, or a friend. As I mentioned earlier, new activities are naturally more fun and exciting. I think it's worth the investment once in a while to try something new and interesting if it keeps you engaged in moving your body regularly. But I also wholeheartedly believe that fitness doesn't always have to be fun! It's too much pressure to always expect you're going to love every single workout. Then it becomes an easy excuse to skip exercise altogether. Instead of avoiding it, reframe exercise and remind yourself of your *Why*. Remember: There are good reasons why exercise matters to you. Use them as motivation and keep searching for routines you enjoy the most.

My client Danielle spent several years trying different types of fitness routines before she started to see a shift in her motivation to move. She got there because she was committed to finding her fitness "fit." Through many attempts she was able to discover her "hate it," "like it," and "love it" routines. She is so much happier with her fitness routines now, and you can be, too.

Roadblock #4: It's Not "Working"

Probably the greatest myth of exercise is the expectation that it leads to weight loss. By and large, we either hope to lose weight or prevent weight gain through exercise. I have had clients tell me outright, "If I don't lose weight, I'm quitting."

(Not a helpful mindset.) Even researchers, who supposedly can control for all types of conditions in studies, are not able to consistently produce long-term weight loss results through exercise. (Trust me, they're trying.)

We all have a friend who lost ten or fifty pounds running, biking, kickboxing, Zumba-ing, or doing the zebra belly dance, but please don't make the mistake of using one example as convincing evidence that it works for everyone. First, you have to account for genetics and size diversity. You are not your friend. You don't know the whole story. And second, we are living creatures, not predictable calorie equations. Well-documented research studies point to the conclusion that exercise alone is poor at efforts to control body weight. One explanation is that exercise increases hunger. You move more and you eat more. Plus, remember the tricky reward system I mentioned in the choice traps in Chapter 1. *Let exercise itself be the reward, not food and drinks you "earned" from physical activity.* Recently, a study attempted to produce weight loss in a group of participants over a ten-month period through significant exercise (the equivalent of running 20 to 30 miles a week); participants only lost one third of the *predicted* weight. Moreover, 25 percent of the participants had zero changes in their weight and 15 to 20 percent actually gained weight (body fat) during the study! Exercise impacts everyone's appearance differently, but does that mean exercise is not effective? No way! All exercise is good for you, but it's unrealistic to use appearance as your most important positive outcome. Maybe it's time for a shift in perspective. There are many health-giving benefits to caring for your body through movement. You don't have to look lean, svelte, shredded, skinny, or cellulite-free to get good results from making a habit out of exercise.

Roadblock #5: It Doesn't Count If It Doesn't Hurt

"No pain, no gain" may be a popular saying among bodybuilders, but my favorite saying with clients is "No pain, no PAIN!" While I am up for physical and mental challenges as part of a well-rounded and fun exercise plan, I'm not up for the idea that your workout sucks if it's not practically killing you. **Moderation is not for wussies. In fact, it's better for you than going to extremes.**

Author and psychologist Michael Otto, PhD, is well known for his research and client work related to the mental health benefits of exercise. One of the reasons he promotes moderate intensity in exercise is that you are more likely to feel confident and optimistic during less strenuous activities. In order to keep coming back for more, your brain needs to make positive mental connections with what you're doing. People who focus solely on strenuous workouts are more likely to become frustrated or discouraged and are less likely to continue their efforts long term. Even running for five minutes a day has health benefits. And if you're a "never gonna run" type of girl—just walk. I dare you to try to stop at five minutes once you've started. Low intensity and low expectations are the perfect recipe for a fun, pain-free workout!

Moderate-intensity movement also helps you avoid doing too much or pushing yourself too hard, which could happen out of desperation to lose weight, tone up quickly, or alter your body. Over-exercising means beating up on your body, not taking care of it.

If the thought of pulling back from intense exercise freaks you out—chances are that's exactly what you need. Have you ever canceled social plans so you could work out or felt like your whole day was ruined because you didn't exercise? If you have any concerns about your motivation for intense exercise, test yourself. Give yourself a week of slowpoke fitness. Take rest days, do a restorative yoga class, or go on a leisurely stroll instead of doing your regular workout.

The Art of Mindful Movement

Moving mindfully means paying attention to how your body feels and noticing as much detail as possible about whatever you're doing. Paying attention to your breathing and trying to clear your mind of outside thoughts puts you fully in touch with the physical and mental benefits of exercise. Checking in with yourself in this way also gives you important information.

There are four components that make up *mindful movement*: Exercise to **rejuvenate your body,** not to exhaust or deplete it. You decide the intensities that feel right to you. Enhance your **mind** and body connection. Don't confuse it. Mindful movement feels like something good you're doing for yourself. You might notice your increased breathing, heart rate, sweating, or other changes during exercise as a way of staying connected. **Alleviate mental and physical stress.** Don't add to it. Approach movement with a sense of ease. New activities or other factors might create some emotional discomfort, but if you stay connected you can observe yourself easing into comfort. **Create pleasure,** not punishment. When you move mindfully, you can observe harsh thoughts and feelings that might harm your well-being.

Spiral Up
ZEN IN MOTION

. . . .

This exercise is intended to help you increase your mindful movement skills. Choose something you already feel comfortable doing, such as walking or another light, outdoor cardio exercise. Set aside more time than normal and make sure your clothing is comfortable and appropriate for the weather. While you are exercising, take time to notice your breath and all of your senses. Try not to change how you breathe or force your body into any specific rhythm. Just let the breath come and go naturally, and notice any changes that happen as you continue walking. Try to incorporate all of your senses into the experience. Make note of the sounds around you: dogs barking, cars going by, people chatting. If judgments or thoughts and opinions come to mind, try to return your attention to your breath. Continue this exercise for the duration of your walk. By doing this, you have essentially given a nice workout to both your body and your brain at the same time. This technique can also be applied to more strenuous or complex activities once you become comfortable with the process.

Whether you're beating up on your body or criticizing your performance, reframe your perspective to one that respects your self-care goals.

This kind of mindful attention can be applied to any form of exercise and will increase your enjoyment. Even if you're just walking, pay attention to posture, keeping your back straight, feeling the flex and release of muscles. Now, if you're thinking you need a distraction so you don't have to think about the pain you're experiencing while you exercise, chances are you're pushing yourself harder than you need to.

Another point worth mentioning is that sometimes, during exercise, we experience sensations that are mildly uncomfortable. Mindful movement can help you become more aware of normal body responses, such as increased heart rate and body temperature or mild burning in your muscles. These physiological reactions are all normal—though I encourage you to take a rest and listen to your body if any significant pain occurs. It is normal to feel mildly sore after learning a new exercise and using muscles that have been out of practice. You may even feel very sore hours or days after a particularly challenging workout. Walking helps muscles recover better than resting. Take an Epsom salt bath, and get a massage or use a foam roller. Your muscles will come back stronger, ready to take on your next movement challenge with gusto.

The most beneficial exercise is the one you do consistently. By practicing mindfulness in your movements and choosing body kindness, I hope you find the sweet spot between challenge and comfort, where the true joy of movement can be found.

Fueling Your Fitness Routines

Fueling your body helps you perform in all areas of life—and your workout routines are no exception. A well-timed meal or snack serves as fuel for your activity; it also helps you perform your best, recover optimally, and get the most out of your exercise. Ideally, meals or snacks should take place thirty to ninety minutes before physical activity. If you're within an hour of a workout, you don't need much; just a piece of fruit or a cup of 100 percent fruit juice or sports drink would do the trick. A mix of foods that provide carbohydrates and proteins will deliver the maximum support for both energy and recovery, i.e., yogurt with granola, oatmeal with peanut butter, egg and avocado toast, smoothies. Sometimes chocolate milk is an upstanding, quick and delicious choice. Don't exercise on empty. Your body and mind will feel the deficit. Respect your body by giving it some fuel for the fitness work you ask it to do.

Discover the Warrior Within

One of the most dramatic changes in my personal fitness mindset happened when I decided to see myself as an athlete. Athletes are strong and powerful. Athletes set and achieve goals that stretch their current abilities. Do something you don't believe you can do—a real challenge that interests you even if you do it only once, like a race. Find a fitness edge that feels challenging in a good way. Take up functional fitness, where you can learn exercises that help you do more in life—like upper body strength to support your passion for gardening, or movements to help build stamina for your upcoming European vacation where you'll do lots of walking and hiking, or take a self-defense class series that teaches you something useful.

My client Hope shared her curiosity about a new, more intense fitness class she had heard about. She wanted to try it but was holding herself back with "What if it's hard, or I can't finish?" We talked about adjustments she could make and benefits of trying the class until she worked up the courage to take the leap. The process of getting there was just as important as anything she may have done once she entered the class. Yes, it was challenging. Yes, she was sore the next day, but she was also energized. She had fun and she felt stronger. With her newfound motivation, Hope became more comfortable challenging herself in other ways, and her entire fitness belief system changed for the better. She learned she was stronger and more capable than she gave herself credit for and that fitness could be fun and challenging at the same time.

BODY KINDNESS REFLECTION: How would you like to enhance your connection to your body through feel-good movement? Describe the good, the bad, and the ugly parts of fitness in your life. Then describe what you want your fitness future to be—in a month and in a year.

"Exercise because you love your body, not because you hate it."
—A body kindness practitioner

Chapter 4

Sleep

······································

The Secret Superpower for Spiraling Up

Philosophy

Sleep is mind-body rejuvenation that helps you become your best—inside and out. There is no substitute. To maximize your energy, positive mood, and healthy body functions, practice good sleep hygiene (self-care habits that support high-quality rest). When you cheat yourself on sleep, your brain's decision-making ability is comparable to a drunk person's. If you don't want to spend your days with the brain of a freshman on a Sunday morning, you'll make sleep a priority. Your body already has built-in mechanisms for getting good sleep and making up for poor sleep. It's a matter of doing what you can to work with these systems and having a body kindness backup plan for when you don't sleep well.

BODY KINDNESS PILLARS
Support Body Kindness
with Rejuvenating Sleep

LOVE: Respect your body by saying "yes" to sleep. Pull away from life in order to recharge yourself for the people and things that matter.

CONNECT: Notice your body's normal, dependable signs of fatigue and allow yourself to stop and rest, or go to sleep.

CARE: Practice regular bedtime rituals to help you unwind and peacefully transition to restful sleep.

Stop the Sleep Shortage

I'm going to go out on a limb and guess that you know from personal experience how sleep patterns can make all the difference in your energy, attitude, and well-being. When you don't sleep enough, the brain fog alone makes you want to take a day off from anything that resembles body kindness—bring on the caffeine and sugar, nix the jog. (Thrive? Yeah, right. It's more like *survive*.) It's hard to be happy, optimistic, and motivated to take care of yourself when you're exhausted. But the good news is you can manage a day of low energy without going on a self-sabotaging downward spiral of poor choices. And your body does a pretty good job helping you make up for a night of not-so-good rest by signaling you to snatch a few extra hours the next night.

Some people have no problem setting and respecting boundaries for their shut-eye. If that's you, keep it up. You'll find ways to enhance the wonderful sleep experience even more, and you'll create a plan for bouncing back in the rare event you feel the consequences of a bad night's sleep. Everyone else (you know who you are) needs to do a better

Spiral Up

Think about how you feel the day after a really good night's sleep. How much easier is it to soar through your day, spiraling up in energy and mood, compared to one or more nights of bad sleep? What words come to mind when you describe the kind of person you act like when you don't get enough shut-eye? Are you cranky? Distracted? Emotional? Mean? (I know I am.) In what ways does your commitment to practicing body kindness help you get the sleep you need? And when your sleep suffers, how does it make it harder for you to eat well, exercise, and roll with stress? Which version of yourself do you want to be, and what are you willing to do to protect your need for good quality sleep?

job at sleeping to pave the way for new, healthful body kindness practice.

There are two primary reasons people don't sleep enough. The first category is about choices and the second category includes a number of physical and mental health problems that can make it difficult to fall asleep or stay asleep. If you're dealing with any sleep-related health issues, improving your daily choices and sleep routines may be part of your treatment plan for getting better rest. But it's important to know that if you are having chronic sleep difficulties, like insomnia or sleep apnea, it may not be something you can fix with a few yoga poses and lavender oil. These are real conditions that need real care. This group also includes parents with kids of any age—I know that getting the sleep you need is not always in your control. On the plus side, we know that exercise and eating well help improve sleep-related conditions and concerns. Be kind to yourself—and if you need help, speak with a health care professional you trust and make sure sleep is part of the conversation.

Most sleep slackers fit into our first poor-sleep category: poor sleep boundaries. They stay up late and then wake up early to a shrill alarm clock jarring them from dreamland. Overbooked and overwhelmed, they designate the wee hours of the night, when they should be sleeping, as the only permissible time to get extra work done—or to be without obligations and relax.

Dilemma of the Sleep Deprived

Five percent of humans possess a genetic mutation that allows them to wake up refreshed and energetic after just six hours of sleep. Everyone else—all 95 percent of us—feel the effects of too little sleep. There's a big difference between a few bad nights of sleep due to living a normal life—and consistently sabotaging your body's need to shut down.

Most of my clients make a U-turn in their sleep patterns once they understand the life-supporting functions of sleep and get a few good nights' rest to feel the difference. In fact, how you feel when you wake in the morning is your best indicator of whether you are getting enough shut-eye. Once you determine that the benefits of good sleep are important to you, you'll get there. It's a matter of paying attention. Your body signals a time to slow things down. As the day goes on, sleepiness sets in. Your master biological clock syncs with the darkness and your brain releases melatonin, a natural sedative that helps ensure sleep is just around the corner. Cortisol, which provides energy, dips at bedtime, and gradually rises again overnight to initiate daytime alertness.

Sleep Science— a Quick Lesson

I'm going to give you a quick sleep science lesson in hopes that understanding more about what your body does during sleep will motivate you to make it a priority. Over the last fifty years, sleep research has exploded, and we are learning that sleep is a busy time for your brain and body to recover from one day and get ready for the next. Generally, sleep occurs in cycles lasting roughly 90 to 120 minutes, and you should complete five cycles per night for maximum benefit. Most people function best during waking hours when they get eight to nine hours of uninterrupted sleep at night.

As you first drift off to sleep, you become disengaged from your surroundings, and you might feel like you are falling or experience a random muscle twitch in one of your legs. These are natural and normal parts of the body's transition into sleep.

Next you enter one of the primary sleep stages—a deep sleep called Slow Wave Sleep (SWS). This is the most restorative sleep you experience. In just twenty minutes, your body is actively rejuvenating on multiple levels—a full-scale daily makeover for your insides. Your immune system, muscles, and tissues are strengthened and repaired, energy is restored, and many essential hormones are released (including the ones responsible for a healthy metabolism). At the same time, your brain's "waste management systems" activate, flushing out the mental garbage of your day. This is your brain's way of clearing unnecessary clutter, making room to help you handle whatever the next day will bring. When I'm tired and my brain feels full but I want to keep working, I like to imagine trash floating around in toxic sludge inside my head and sleep is the magical force that sucks it all away!

After this initial phase of deep sleep, your body enters twenty minutes of Rapid Eye Movement (REM) sleep. This is when your eyes dart back and forth beneath closed eyelids. If you've ever stared at someone experiencing this, it can be quite an unsettling thing to see! While this is happening, your muscles actually become paralyzed, so you can't even move. Your brain activity is very high during REM, and this is when dreams take place. In the divine wisdom of human creation, I think it's for our own safety and the safety of our bedmates that we're not able to move while we dream. Who knows what I might have done that night I dreamt my husband ran off with the nanny!

And that crazy dream about losing all your teeth, frantically trying to find them, and then racing to the dentist because you have a date in an hour is part of an important psychological process. While you're dreaming, your brain is busy creating memories. It filters real-life experiences and decides what you will learn and remember. Whether you want to be a better swimmer, sewer, or singer, your "sleep lesson" is just as important as your "awake lesson." When you dream, your brain is learning what you practiced so it can get better at controlling your muscles. Babies who are approaching a movement milestone actually practice while they sleep. Many parents have witnessed an emerging crawler squirming around the crib at night, fast asleep, right before becoming fully mobile. **Dreams are also closely connected to our emotional health. By processing negative emotions, we often begin to feel more positive again and wake up with a fresh perspective.** Ever wonder where the phrase "Why don't you sleep on it?" came from? I'm sure we all have a story of a kerfuffle that could have been avoided had we just paused, gone to bed, let our brains do some work, and woken up with a more rational perspective.

YOUR BODY ON SLEEP

WHEN YOU GET ENOUGH GOOD SLEEP, YOUR BODY
RESPONDS IN WAYS THAT ENHANCE YOUR HEALTH.

BRAIN
You have better
decision-making,
focus, concentration,
memory, and reaction
time. You're more
likely to make choices
that support your
health goals, showing
self-control when
temptation strikes.

FACE
Your skin
is more
supple and
hydrated.

EYES
They are
naturally white
and not bloodshot.
You're less likely to
have dark circles
under your
eyes.

APPETITE
Hormones that regulate
your metabolism, hunger,
and appetite are working
optimally so you're more
likely to make feel-good
choices.

HEART
A good night's sleep fosters emotional resilience. You feel optimistic and ready for the day. You're in a better place to deal with drama and have compassion for others—and yourself!

MUSCLES
They're fueled up and ready to move you any which way to carry you through work and play.

IMMUNE SYSTEM
You are stockpiled and ready to fight any virus or bacteria that dares enter your body.

How Bad Is Bad Sleep?

Lack of sleep is like torture. There's a reason they use sleep deprivation as a tactic to break down war criminals. Without proper sleep, you can turn into a "junk food junkie," searching for your next hit of sugar-, salt-, or carb-laden food to survive the day. All it takes is one night for you to feel the negative effects of bad sleep and you're on a downward spiral of poor choices, one after the other. "Screw it, I don't care, shut up—I need it, this sucks" are the grumblings of a droopy-eyed, disheveled, sleep-deprived zombie.

When your brain doesn't have the chance to recharge by sleeping, you make unclear, irrational decisions. There's even a name for it: mild prefrontal dysfunction. It's kind of like temporary brain damage. Being mildly but chronically sleep deprived, edging out a few hours here and there out of habit, is the cognitive equivalent of a blood alcohol level of 0.1 percent—drunk. Research shows that missing just 1.5 hours of sleep can reduce your daytime alertness by 32 percent. Based on this information, most of us could be deemed unsafe for driving, including all the sleep-deprived parents carting minivans full of children across town.

When you are short on sleep, you're an emotional live wire, reacting even more negatively to the little things that don't go your way. To add insult to injury, the part of your brain that causes you to rage is hyperactive when you are short on sleep. I have clear memories of eye-popping, nostril-flaring anger toward my (very funny) husband for making jokes when he was in a good mood and I was fumbling around on three hours of sleep.

Sleep-deprived people are less friendly and empathetic, and they lack the ability to praise personal achievement or even notice when something good happens that day. Some experts recommend we avoid challenging and potentially frustrating tasks and even limit social interaction when we are very short on sleep. But when hiding out isn't an option, try to be kind to yourself and shift your expectations. Instead of pushing harder and doubling up on espresso to work through the fatigue, try to get as much water and movement as possible to give yourself natural boosts throughout the day.

Create a Sleep Sanctuary to Fall Asleep Happy

You know that feeling when you walk into a great spa or fancy hotel room and you just know the experience is going to be luxurious? That's how you should feel when you enter your bedroom. Here's how the most effective sleepers set bedroom boundaries to find their sleep "sweet spot."

Spiral Up

A BODY KINDNESS SLEEP SCAN

* On a scale of 1 to 5, how satisfied are you with the amount of sleep you get most nights?

* What are some of the challenges you face that make good, restful sleep elusive?

* How is not getting enough sleep affecting you during waking hours?

* How much do you rely on caffeine and alcohol to help you cope with skewed sleeping patterns?

* Start a sleep diary: Track your sleeping habits for a week, including the time you go to bed and wake up, how you feel upon waking, how long it takes you to fall asleep, the number of times you wake in the night, what you do while awake, and how long it takes you to fall back asleep.

Information you gather from a sleep scan can help you set goals to improve the quality of your sleep. Even better, should you choose to speak to your doctor, therapist, or a sleep specialist about your concerns, this information will make it easier for them to help you.

RESERVE YOUR ROOM FOR SLEEP AND SEX. Get rid of anything in the room that does not promote these activities. Vibrators can stay (obviously), but TVs are out. Keep only the things you really need in your bedroom.

MAKE SURE YOUR BED IS COMFORT-ABLE AND CLEAN. If your mattress isn't comfortable, or if it's older than about seven years, make an investment in your sleep quality with a new mattress. This isn't a splurge; it's a necessity, and good sleep has enough financial benefits to help justify the cost. Wash your bedding every week to prevent the natural accumulation of allergens and dust mites, which can lead to poor quality sleep.

GIVE YOURSELF A BEDTIME. Attempt to go to bed early enough to be asleep for about eight hours. Stop using any blue-light emitting screens at least an hour before bed. Blue light delays your body's release of the melatonin that lulls you to sleep.

KEEP YOUR NIGHTSTAND CLEAR AND ORGANIZED. All you really need is a glass of water and a book—a real paper book—or a journal and pen. NO screens. Yes, this includes your smartphone. If it acts as your alarm clock, keep it on the other side of the room.

GET YOUR ROOM DARK, COOL, AND CALM. Make sure your bedroom is dark when you go to bed. Use black-out curtains if you need them. Keep your room on the cool side and use blankets. Heat delays your body's sleep cycle. Place a drop of lavender essential oil on your temples or pillow, or mix it with water in a diffuser or a spray bottle. It's known for its calming effect.

ADD WHITE NOISE. If noises awaken you in the night, use a fan or a white noise machine. If you like falling asleep to music but it occasionally wakes you up, set a timer so it turns off automatically.

TURN IT DOWN BEFORE TURNING IN. Give yourself an extra hour before bedtime to relax and unwind. If you're feeling anxious or stressed, write down your thoughts and come up with ways to alleviate your concerns, which you can implement the following day. End your night with relaxing deep breathing rituals or restorative yoga poses to help you get into the sleep zone.

DRESS FOR THE OCCASION. Do your pajamas make you happy? I love wearing my birthday suit to bed! Wear what you love the best, not just any ratty tank top and sweat pants—unless that's what you love to wear.

How to Spiral Up with Sleep, Food, and Fitness

The relationships among sleep, eating habits, and exercise choices are multidirectional. They all have the potential to enhance one another. A positive choice in one area can create an upward spiral, increasing the chances of making a good choice in another area.

Optimal sleep improves your metabolism, energy, and mood. When you get enough sleep, your body releases adequate levels of a hormone called leptin, which regulates your metabolism and suppresses your appetite. Leptin and its counterpart, ghrelin, are usually secreted at specific intervals throughout the night. Ideally, you're asleep well before these hormones are released and you stay asleep so you can get enough of them. When you sleep well, these hormones allow your hunger and fullness signals to function properly, making it easier to choose foods that make you feel good and add to your energy reserves.

In general, healthful eating and good sleep go hand in hand. Certain foods may help you fall asleep because their nutrients can kick your body's sleep patterns into gear. Melatonin, nature's sleeping pill, is key in maintaining your circadian rhythm. A few foods, like tart cherry juice, have melatonin. Our bodies are very good at releasing melatonin and serotonin (a relaxation hormone) when we provide the right nutrients. The B vitamins help produce serotonin and melatonin from carbohydrate-rich foods (low-carb eaters be warned!). The minerals calcium and magnesium are also important to sleep. Foods with sleep-inducing powers won't always put you into a drowsy state if you have them in the morning or afternoon. Just having the nutrients in your system is enough.

If you are the kind of person who likes a bedtime snack or you find yourself hungry a bit before bed, the food choices you make can strengthen your ability to fall asleep. Any food you eat before bedtime should be small in portion size to avoid discomfort or digestive problems. Be careful about food and beverage choices that can interfere with good sleep, like alcohol or anything with caffeine, including chocolate. If you're already tired, skip the snack and head to bed. My clients who complain of bored and mindless eating late at night are often just tired and avoiding sleep. Ask yourself, "Could I go to sleep now or am I hungry enough that I won't be able to sleep?" If you're not sure (and tired brains can get easily confused on this), then choose a light, healthful snack. If you're not interested in a healthful snack, that's a good clue that you're not really hungry.

Foods to Help You Sleep

Try some of these snack pairings for an evening concoction to take you to la-la land with a happy belly. Keep your portions around fist-sized, such that your belly still feels comfortable, and eat at least an hour before you want to fall asleep.

A "MOCKTAIL" OF tart cherry juice and warm chamomile tea will deliver a dose of melatonin from the cherries and glycine from the chamomile, relaxing nerves and muscles and acting as a mild sedative.

CHEESE AND CRACKERS (hold the wine) will provide you with calcium and carbohydrates to help you sleep.

HUMMUS AND PRETZELS. This creamy-and-crunchy snack will help your body make serotonin and melatonin.

OATMEAL MADE WITH milk and topped with pistachios, wheat germ, and dried tart cherries provides several key sleep nutrients.

MAC-N-CHEESE. Hello, comfort food! Cheese and carbohydrates in the evening will make your brain and belly relaxed and happy.

PREMIUM ICE CREAM. Go for a small scoop of the good stuff to satisfy a sweet craving and give you just enough carbohydrates and calcium to nod off.

OR CREATE YOUR own snack list from these types of foods. Just make sure you feel calm and comfortable with what you're eating.

Eating Your Way Out of a Sleep Deficit?

What kinds of foods do you think are the drugs of the sleep-deprived? (Hint: They're not fruits or vegetables.) What we typically call comfort foods—because they are, well, comforting—can also cause some of the most intense food cravings you may ever experience in your life. These tend to be foods that are sources of quick energy—foods that provide sugars, fats, and sodium. These kinds of foods are palate pleasing and satiate our impulsive animal brain, which has a one-track mind—energy, energy, energy. While it may feel like your body is conspiring against you, it's actually trying to help you get out of an energy pickle primarily caused by your sleep deficit.

Your brain releases hormones that support a normally functioning metabolism at various stages of sleep, late into the night and in the very early morning. When you get fewer than seven hours of sleep your appetite hormones are dysregulated. Your levels of the "hunger" hormone, ghrelin (which slows metabolism and increases appetite), are higher than usual, and you don't have enough of the hormone leptin (which speeds metabolism and suppresses appetite) because you woke up before your brain could finish releasing all the leptin into your body.

The second problem in this craving chaos is that your cells are tired and not doing their job. They have trouble absorbing glucose (your main source of energy). Your brain perceives this as "Hey, we're all starving around here, give us some food and we'll give you some energy." Your brain then increases your cravings and desire for quick energy (the comfort foods). And because your

Spiral Up
SWEET DREAMS
WITH GENTLE MOVEMENT

Restorative yoga is a short sequence of poses supported by props that allow you to completely relax and rest. You hold poses like gentle twists, forward folds, and easy back bends for several minutes at a time, while breathing comfortably. Restorative yoga is based on the teachings of yoga guru B.K.S. Iyengar.

Yoga nidra or "yogic sleep" allows you to teeter between awake and sleep consciousness, similar to a guided meditation. You follow a practitioner's guidance over audio, gradually bringing your focus inward, often scanning your body while breathing calmly, and entering a completely relaxed state. The last few minutes of yoga class, particularly the savasana (corpse pose), are a form of yoga nidra. There are many books and free resources to help you with these practices.

Qigong is a dynamic meditation for health maintenance, healing, and increasing vitality. Instead of counting sheep, try this simple relaxation exercise to help you sleep by drawing energy out of your head and directing it to your lower abdomen. By shifting your focus away from distracting thoughts, you'll rest more easily. To start, lie comfortably on your back. Place your hands on your lower belly, about an inch below your belly button. Begin to make large, slow circles in a clockwise direction over your lower belly, keeping your hands in light contact with the skin. The circles should be slow—about four full seconds for each revolution. Eventually you should notice your mind becoming calmer as you shift your focus from your head to your belly. Remember, just like any new exercise, this takes practice. Try not to force yourself to stop thinking, as that is rarely helpful. Instead, simply observe the movement of your thoughts without judgment. Eventually your mind will begin to calm down.

rational decision-making and self-control are diminished in your lack-of-sleep stupor, it's way too easy for you to perceive these signals as something real and to feel powerless against the craving. You "give in" and get the dopamine rush that says "great job, do it again," and the day goes on, one poor choice at a time.

If you're wondering whether lack of sleep could explain recent weight gain or difficulty with weight loss, it depends. Certainly if you take into account the hormone imbalances and food cravings, energy too low for exercise, and overall lack of excitement about sticking to health goals, you can see the downward spiral right there. You don't need a diet, sugar detox, or calorie-counting plan. Sleep is the antidote to a lack of sleep. And until you catch up on your *Z*'s, don't let your food choices be "there's nothing I can do about it" excuses for poor sleep. Be tired and make the food choices that are in line with your ideas of body kindness. **You can choose to satisfy a craving without going overboard.** Remember the three-legged stool from Chapter 2? Be hungry, make balanced food choices, and savor what you eat. Keep in mind that eating well will energize you even if you did not sleep well, which may be the boost you need to stick to your workout *and* get a good night's sleep.

Getting good sleep helps ensure you will have the physical energy and desire to pursue enjoyable exercise during the day. In addition, regular exercise reduces the amount of time it takes to fall asleep

and helps you have a more restful sleep. One study showed that people sleep significantly better with at least 150 minutes of exercise a week. And contrary to popular belief, you don't need to skip exercise in the evening. The relaxation and calm you feel after exercise supports better sleep. You might consider gentler forms of movement later in the evening, like walking, yoga, or meditation.

Sleep is one of the strongest predictors of whether or not we eat well and exercise. As women, many of us are willing to cut into sleep for the needs of others or for the sake of "me time." If you fall into this category along with me, then it's time to fix our schedules and start protecting our sleep! There has to be a way to take care of our jobs, our families, and ourselves within sixteen hours of wakefulness. Otherwise something's got to give—and it will be our brains, bodies, and sanity unless we start taking sleep more seriously.

I'm not saying you have to go to bed at eight o'clock every night for the rest of your life. But please, if you insist on missing sleep, at least make sure it's for something you really care about. Many of my clients tell me they stay up late because it's the only time they get to themselves all day. But when I ask what they are doing with that time, they admit to binge-watching Netflix, sneaking into the ice cream, and mindlessly saving Pinterest projects they'll never complete. So my next question is: "Is this *really* what you want to do with

Spiral Up

MY BODY KINDNESS
BOUNCE BACK PLAN

Spend an hour or so thinking about what you usually do when you don't sleep well and what you would like to do differently. Then write a kind letter of commitment to your future sleep-deprived self in your body kindness journal, to be read when needed as a reminder to take better care of yourself. Something along the lines of:

Dear zombie . . . I'm sorry you feel like crap. We just have to get through the day. I'm committed to helping you make as many good choices as possible so you can enjoy better sleep tonight. Together we are going to take care of you and tackle the day with a smile. Here's what I will do for you today. . . .

Make your self-care decisions when you're well rested, so that when you are tired, you don't need to waste precious brain energy on negative thinking or poor decision-making. You can act like the well-rested person you want to be even if you feel like you're in *Night of the Living Dead*.

your alone time?" The typical response is "Not really, but there's nothing else to do at midnight." If this sounds familiar to you, I don't think you have a sleep problem or a self-care problem—you have a priority problem. Remember the two opposing choice options: short- and long-term reward. Sleep is part of the delayed reward that is more likely to help you create a better life. Sleep is more likely the way to be good to your body in this moment. Tomorrow, you'll thank yourself for the sleep tonight.

Another thing to consider is the length of time it takes to complete your nightly routines. If you tend to dawdle around, getting ready for tomorrow until it's way past bedtime, then decide on an earlier "get ready for bed" time. This means if you want to be asleep by ten thirty, you may need to start wrapping up the day at nine thirty.

Eventually most people who don't get enough sleep at night will develop poor sleep habits (TV in bed, nighttime binge eating, etc.) or irregular sleep patterns (oversleeping, long daytime naps) to compensate. We begin to think this is "just how we are" when in actuality these habits and behavior patterns are red flags telling us that our body and brain are chronically tired.

If you are among the millions of Americans who aren't sleeping and eating well, your lack of willpower isn't to blame, and the solution probably isn't in a prescription bottle. The first place to look for answers is your pillow. You need to fix your sleep. Sleep is essential for your body to help regulate energy levels and appetite, making your body the healthy machine it's intended to be. Trying to reach baseline health goals while getting insufficient sleep is like trying to fix a broken leg with a Band-Aid.

BOUNCING BACK FROM A BAD NIGHT'S SLEEP WITH BODY KINDNESS

EAT WELL. Energize your body the best you can with delicious, nutritious foods you can rely on to make you feel more energetic.

HYDRATE. Hydrate. Hydrate.

MOVE. Even if you don't feel up for a workout, consider any way of moving that you might find pleasurable. Keep in mind that exercise boosts mood and will help you sleep better.

REST DURING THE DAY TO POWER UP. If this option is available to you, take the time for a catnap or rest to let your brain do a little housekeeping. If your body is telling you it needs rest, do your best to listen. Lock your office door if you need to and take a power nap with your head on your desk. Just don't forget to set an alarm!

AVOID BIG DECISIONS AND TOUGH CONVERSATIONS. Observe negative thoughts but don't react. Remind yourself that it's sleep deprivation talking and reach for the easiest meaningful choice until you feel calmer and more rested.

ADOPT AN "I CAN HANDLE IT" ATTITUDE. Fatigue is a feeling caused by lack of sleep. Keeping this in mind can help you maintain emotional balance. Your body is working just fine. Continue making choices that support your body kindness goals despite the urge to crash into a downward spiral.

BE A POLLYANNA TODAY. Don't necessarily fake it, but a positive outlook can help boost your tolerance of the bad, and finding the silver lining will help your resilience. Seek out positive people and purposely choose activities that will boost your spirits.

How to Fall Asleep More Easily

So, what's keeping us up at night and what can we do to change it? Stress is the number one cause of sleep difficulties. Nearly 50 percent of people with occasional insomnia report lying awake at night due to stress. In our 24/7, technology-driven world, the lines between home and work, sleeping and waking have become blurred. Our to-do lists are too long and our calendars are overflowing, so we nudge precious minutes and hours off our sleep each night to compensate. Technology allows us to work across time zones, late into the evening, and when we're finally done with work, there's always TV and social media to keep us going until the wee hours of the morning.

CREATE A SLEEP-INDUCING, STRESS-BUSTING, AND CALMING BEDTIME RITUAL

MAKE A LIST of five nonscreen activities that bring you calm and make you feel good. Some ideas are listening to gentle music, making a phone call to a friend, writing letters, walking the dog, or planning your outfit for the next day.

SPEND SOME EXTRA TIME IN QUIET SOLITUDE. Follow a guided meditation, practice yoga nidra, or put on instrumental music. Begin to wind down your thoughts.

PAMPER YOURSELF. Instead of just falling into bed, take your time washing your face and brushing your teeth, put on a clean T-shirt or pajamas, and massage your feet and hands with scented lotions.

HAVE A BOOK OF POETRY, PRAYERS, OR MEDITATIONS ON YOUR BEDSIDE TABLE and read them nightly. The familiar words will become a natural sleep inducer as your brain associates them with rest and relaxation. Mary Oliver and Rumi are great for this.

BREATHE ON

Thank goodness we can breathe without even thinking about it. But we often take this life force for granted and miss out on the truly powerful impact a few deep breaths can have on our mind, body, and spirit. Breathing is key to relaxation and is also a low-cost, no-risk way to improve sleep. The following are some of my favorite body kindness ideas for bringing focus to your breath. When practiced often, the benefits of deep breathing multiply and strengthen. Start small and increase over time. In as little as five minutes, these activities can create a sense of calm, decrease your heart rate, and stabilize your mood.

ENERGY SLUMP, BUT IT'S NOT TIME FOR BED?

If you're tired but it's hours before a realistic bedtime, this exercise will give your brain a break without taking a nap.

Close your eyes and take a few deep breaths, allowing your belly to rise and fall. On the inhale, fill your belly like a balloon. When you exhale, imagine all the air flowing quickly out of the balloon as your stomach deflates.

TIRED AND READY TO SLEEP? TRY 4-7-8 BREATHING.

This is particularly good when your mind is wandering or you can't seem to calm down stressful thoughts. Inhale four counts, hold seven counts, and exhale eight counts. You're essentially exercising your brain's relaxation response, and the more you challenge it, the stronger it will become!

Lying in bed, start with a few long, slow, deep breaths, without trying to control the exact timing. Just inhale and exhale. Relax your jaw, tongue, and mouth. Release any effort to clench or tighten your face. Begin with a complete exhale through your mouth. Close your mouth and inhale through your nose for a count of four. Now hold your breath for seven counts, then follow with an eight-count *whoosh* exhale through the mouth. Repeat this five times in a row . . . if you are still awake.

Meditation, guided imagery, deep breathing exercises, and progressive muscle relaxation (tensing and relaxing your muscles) can also counter anxiety and racing thoughts to help you fall asleep and stay asleep.

Sink into the bed: Starting with your toes, tighten each muscle of your body as you inhale deeply. Release the muscles as you exhale and imagine that part of your body sinking deeply into the bed. Repeat this for each muscle group from your legs, butt, and stomach, all the way up through your chest, shoulders, neck, head, and face.

Visualize colors: Imagine yourself in a calm, relaxing place, then imagine the colors green and blue appearing when you inhale. Watch the colors move around in your happy space. With your exhale, imagine releasing the color red, or negative emotions: anger, frustration, and the like.

How to Stay Asleep More Easily

Whether it's the loud snoring coming from the other side of the bed or the pitter-patter of little feet down the hall, there are many reasons we find it hard to sleep through the night. But once you realize how important sleep is to everyone's health and sanity, it becomes easier to take the necessary steps to overcome sleep obstacles. If your partner snores, encourage him or her to talk with a physician about it, because chances are you aren't the only one experiencing negative consequences from the noise and there might be a solution. Some couples report success with earplugs, sleep positioning devices, pillows, and white noise machines. Sleeping in another room works, too. It doesn't have to be all the time, but when you *really* need to sleep, there's nothing better than a wall between you and the snorer. In her book *The Sleep Revolution*, Arianna Huffington encourages the different rooms approach if you or your partner struggles with good sleep or if you have different sleep habits: "Perhaps it's time to reclaim the term *sleeping around* to refer not to sex but to finding a place to get the sleep we need."

If you wake up and have difficulty going back to sleep, stay in bed except to pee or get a drink of water. Better yet, keep water at your bedside. **Resting in bed, even if you're not sleeping, is still beneficial to the body.** This can also help reduce the anxiety of not being able to sleep and may naturally lead you back into a sleep pattern. Do breath work, meditations, or visualizations to calm yourself, especially when you wake up and start worrying about all the sleep you are losing. Keep the alarm clock out of sight! The anxiety associated with falling back to sleep is reinforced each time you check the time and start counting down the minutes until sunrise.

If you feel like you've been awake for longer than twenty minutes (without checking the clock) and still can't fall back to sleep, then experts suggest you get up and participate in a brief, non-stimulating activity until you feel tired again. This doesn't mean go online, check email, or watch TV. Read a book of poetry, or go for boredom and read a textbook or an instruction manual. I have one client who swears that folding a load of laundry in the middle of the night is just enough mindless effort to remind her brain and body she'd rather be in bed asleep.

You can also try a sleep mantra, which is a phrase or sentence that you repeat to yourself as soon as you become aware of wakefulness during the night. The more often you do this the easier it will become. It could be "Good night, brain, let's talk about this in the morning." Maybe it's a familiar prayer or the words to a song. Once you commit to this strategy, try it right away anytime you wake up over the next few weeks, saying the words over and over again whenever you want to fall back asleep. If your thoughts wander (and they probably will), no problem, just watch them go by and bring yourself back to the familiar words, repeating the mantra gently to yourself.

BODY KINDNESS REFLECTION: Open your journal and record your thoughts and feelings about sleep. In what ways do your current sleep habits enhance body kindness? In what ways would you like to improve your sleep?

> "Sleep is that golden chain that ties health and our bodies together."
>
> —Thomas Dekker

Part Two

How You Feel

....

Embrace Your Emotions

Chapter 5

All Feelings Matter

How Bad Feelings Are Good for You

Philosophy

All feelings, even negative ones, are actually important to your well-being because they offer guidance for decision-making. Sometimes when you feel bad you end up making decisions you really don't want to make—sabotaging your best body kindness efforts and thrusting yourself into a downward spiral. Mastering how you handle your emotions is key to transforming your health habits. Once you begin to understand that all your emotions have a purpose, you can learn how to take better care of yourself and practice body kindness no matter how you feel.

BODY KINDNESS PILLARS
Embracing Your Emotions

LOVE: Loving yourself includes granting yourself permission to feel the full spectrum of emotions for a healthy, happy, and meaningful life.

CONNECT: Feel how your emotions manifest in your mind and body and use this information to guide yourself toward self-care.

CARE: Make choices that allow a sense of calm, ease, or peacefulness when you're feeling negative emotions. Remain committed to taking care of yourself.

The "I Can't" Story

"I'm not sure you're going to be able to help me," she said. "It's not you—it's just that I already know so much about healthful eating and exercise. I've been to nutritionists before. I've tried and I just keep failing. I know what I should be doing—or not doing. I just don't do it. I can't do it. And I don't know why."

Every person I have ever helped has some variation of the "I can't do it" story. Interestingly, something in them believes change is possible because they're in my office, but the first thing they admit is having a low opinion of their ability to change. It's only when they see themselves succeeding, making the choices they want to make, that they start believing they *can* change.

What if I told you the most likely reason people don't achieve goals is because of the voices in their heads? (For many of us, there is more than one!) The most effective way to overcome mental roadblocks and build lasting habits is to acknowledge the negative thoughts you're hearing from yourself—and then go do what you need to do anyway! Pause for a second and really consider that. Imagine observing your thoughts, feelings, and beliefs, no matter how horrible they are, saying "Hello, I see you," and

Spiral Up

W hat would your life be like if you could feel only positive emotions? How would you appreciate what "happy" feels like if you were never sad? How would you know being too hard on yourself was wrong if you couldn't feel hurt by your negative thoughts? In what ways can getting in touch with your feelings help you practice body kindness?

then making the rational body kindness choice anyway. Whether you're thinking "sounds interesting, I'll try it" or "this will never work," it doesn't matter. Those thoughts are just words—a story you're telling yourself. And the story does not have to define your next decision.

This is the essence of how you will take back your power of choice and build *psychological flexibility*—the ability to think about how you feel and make body kindness choices even when it's difficult to do so. It's the most joyful way to create new habits because, for once, it involves nonaction! You simply do not allow your unhelpful thoughts—that made-up story in your head—to influence your choices. It's more effective than trying to "just think positive" or using self-affirmation approaches because those activities can feel phony when you pretend like your thoughts and feelings aren't real. Passively observing your thoughts is more effective than challenging your thoughts, asking if they're true or trying to make them go away. Who cares if the thought is true or not? It's just a bunch of words—nothing more. You can still make body kindness choices, regardless of what you're thinking and feeling.

Don't Take the Bait

Thoughts are constantly swirling around in your head. Like a radio with a broken dial, you can't turn them off. Helpful thoughts are constructive and motivate you toward self-improvement decisions. Even if a thought makes you feel uncomfortable—like reminding you of a goal—it can be helpful if it's compassionate. "I know you're tired and stressed, but your exercise plan is important to you. Exercise will help you deal with the stress." Any thought you have that does not serve to make your life better or help you accomplish your goals deserves the "unhelpful" label. "I don't have time, motivation, or willpower. I have failed before, I'll fail again," etc., etc. These are all forms of "I can't do it!" Unhelpful thoughts are obstacles, judgments,

Spiral Up
MAKE FRIENDS
WITH YOUR FEELINGS

When something's not right and you don't know how to act, start with PACT.

PRESENCE. Be aware. What's happening right now that matters to me, and will my thoughts lead me to positive change?

ACCEPTANCE. No matter how I'm feeling, it's OK to be here right now.

CHOICE. Make a decision. What choice option helps me create a better life? What's one thing I can do now to spiral up?

TAKE ACTION. Follow through on the choice with committed action. The sooner the better.

Become more mindful of your high-intensity emotional triggers and likely ways you'll respond with the *feelings* sentence.

"_____ happened and I feel _____. I want to _____ but instead I will _____."

First blank = the trigger
Identify an event that you think is influencing your thoughts and feelings. "I don't know" is a valid answer.

Second blank = your emotions
Name at least one way you feel right now. Usually a negative event or thought is followed by a negative emotion. Remember, even bad feelings can be beneficial.

Third blank = the automatic response
This may be listening to the negative thought, avoiding an emotion, or any behavior you have learned to do when certain thoughts and feelings arise. These responses are unhelpful and do not get you closer to your body kindness goals.

Fourth blank = a helpful action
This is what you will do instead of the unhelpful urge. You can name one action to take or several, just don't delay. The quicker you take action the better you will feel.

comparisons, and predictions, serving no purpose but to keep you stuck and afraid of taking action.

Think of a few words to describe how unhelpful thoughts make you feel. Based on what you're thinking and feeling, imagine what you're likely to do. Are you really more likely to practice body kindness in this mindset? No way, Jose! Thoughts can have a powerful impact on what you do. Suddenly it doesn't matter what you know about taking care of yourself. Unhelpful thoughts work you up emotionally. You can often feel it in your body—fast heartbeat, tightness in your chest, tension in your muscles, clenched jaw. You're like a hungry fish. You take the bait, get hooked on negative thinking, and are stuck struggling with all this bad energy. Your very next decision will not be calm and rational if you're entangled in negativity. But the beauty of all of this is that you don't have to get hooked at all. Instead, make a PACT with yourself: Presence, Acceptance, Choice, Take action.

PACT is a mindfulness practice. The goal is to become aware of what's happening and curious about how you can help yourself. You practice accepting whatever is going on instead of struggling with it or ignoring it. When you get yourself out of the thought trap, you are free to make a meaningful choice and take immediate action without wasting any more brainpower. PACT offers a strategy to deal with complex and confusing emotions while saving your energy for what matters most.

When my clients learn PACT and start practicing it, some of them tell me they find mindfulness challenging. "When I was numb, it was easier. I just disconnected and went on automatic pilot." Don't be surprised if this brings up things that are unsettling for you. If you find it difficult to engage with your thoughts and feelings, remind yourself that this is what it feels like to fully experience life. You're noticing what's happening and dealing with it. If the upward spirals don't happen immediately, they will start soon.

Feeling Good and Feeling Bad
Are Good for You

Happy, sad, good, bad—from melancholy to morose, cheerful to joyous, and everything in between—human beings are a virtual whirlwind of fleeting emotions. When you notice you feel good, you tend to identify with the state of happiness. You experience a sense of satisfaction, pleasure, gladness, and gratification. For the most part, feeling good feels "right," like it's where you're supposed to be. You're spiraling up with energy and radiating it out to the world around you. Body kindness can be pretty effortless when you feel good. In contrast, feeling bad can feel "wrong." You generally don't like living in Gloomville and you're looking for the fastest exit out of there. In a way, that's a good thing. It keeps you out of depression and drives you toward more positive emotions as your default state of being. Feeling negative emotions is your body's way of telling you, "Something is wrong and I need your attention." When you experience a low mood, motivation for practicing body kindness will naturally be deflated, and that's OK. You aren't meant to feel happy all the time. The more experienced you become at recognizing all of your emotions, the better equipped you will be to make body kindness choices as you navigate the ups and downs and highs and lows of life. It's important to have the mindset that "When I feel bad I am not helpless." You can always use the power of choice to practice body kindness.

Embracing all your emotions may be the most important aspect of practicing body kindness, especially if you can relate to coping with your emotions in ways that don't feel like body kindness—such as emotional overeating, binge eating, depriving yourself of food, excessive drinking, isolating yourself from friends and family, skipping workouts, trash-talking yourself, or neglecting your mind and body in other ways. Bad feelings don't have to lead to choices you'll regret later. In fact, practicing body kindness when you feel bad is a fast track to spiraling up and feeling better faster.

Part of the function of emotions is providing you with information to make choices. Brain scientist and author Jill Bolte Taylor argues that, biologically, humans are *feeling creatures* who *also* think. You are constantly scanning your surroundings using all your senses, and then your brain attempts to make meaning out of information you collect. You make judgments about what's going on based on your perception—a combination of your thoughts and feelings—not necessarily facts. In the most basic sense, your thoughts and feelings are trying to be helpful—"I am safe" or "I am in danger." Your biological system is set up to alert you to dangers so you can respond to them appropriately. The trepidation you feel before crossing a busy street, for instance, helps keep you safe. The pain of negative emotions should communicate to you, "I don't like feeling this way. I need to take action." But if you perceive your negative emotions as dangerous territory, you can become compelled to avoid feeling them altogether by numbing your pain. Every time negative emotions arise, you want to run. It's in the running from pain that rational choices go down the tubes. When you believe bad feelings are beneficial, you don't need to run. If you can engage with them head-on, even when you're afraid, you will better understand their purpose and you'll come up with resourceful decisions on what to do next, if anything at all. Don't disown the feeling. You may not like it. But when you reflect on negative feelings through a body kindness lens, running, numbing, and avoidance are replaced with self-compassion and self-care. As soon as you notice you're entangled in unhelpful thoughts or downward spiraling, just stop whatever it is you're doing and start paying attention. Go through the PACT exercise or complete the feelings sentence. Get curious about what's happening and make a decision that gets you spiraling up.

Visualize the Waves in a Storm and Go Surfing

I love the water. I love the glasslike appearance of lakes and the massive ocean waves that crash on the North Shore of Hale'iwa, Hawaii. Like the sea, emotions can be rough and stormy. Conjure up the image of waves in a storm, observe their strength and power, feel that helplessness during the storm, and then notice that the storm passes and the waves go back to normal. When you're in the middle of a difficult thoughts-and-feelings storm, it's helpful to know that the feelings and urges will come and go without you needing to run or chase them away. Just watch them. Call them out: "It's stormy. Big waves." Bring your mind to a place where it can color that picture. This act alone is a way to redirect your thoughts and attention. Visualize yourself riding out the storm. Let PACT show you the way to safety.

Can you trust that this emotional storm will pass? How can you practice body kindness during the storm? One well-studied technique is called *surfing the urge*, a metaphor for handling impulsive triggers. You ride the wave, so to speak, when you're experiencing an urge to do something you don't want to do. Instead of reaching for food, alcohol, or cigarettes, jump up on your board, hang on, and boogie your way back to shore. It may sound corny to think that your mind can power you through a difficult challenge. There's a magical shift that happens when you try these things and you actually see yourself taking back control of your actions. You visualize yourself making it through the storm, surfing the urges, and when you do make it through, the sense of accomplishment spirals you up and you really start to believe, more than ever, "I got this."

Connection is a core body kindness pillar. Connecting to your feelings on a regular basis, not just when it's stormy, is the most effective way to establish habits that stand the test of time. Once you decide that taking care of yourself is a priority, it becomes part of your job to pay attention to how you feel each day. The goal is to get in touch with your thoughts and feelings, raise your awareness, and then make micro-adjustments based on your responses to questions such as "What feeling have I been experiencing the most recently?" (positive or negative), and then dig a little deeper: "When did I start feeling this way? Do I know what prompted it?" If it's a positive emotion, think about how you can get in touch with it more often. If you are trying to overcome a negative feeling, ask yourself what you would do for a friend who felt this way. Do the same for yourself. It's empowering to realize that even our scariest emotions can serve a helpful purpose when it comes to honoring body kindness.

The more comfortable you become with experiencing all your emotions, the more confident you will be in your body kindness practice. You'll see that even when it's not easy, it's possible to be good to yourself. The practice of mindfulness is the path toward psychological flexibility and building your skills to observe thoughts and feelings without letting them control your response. Anything you do to improve mindfulness—any form of meditation, relaxation, focusing, observing, and engaging with life and the world around you—is beneficial. Practice it regularly, in good times as well as in bad. Then it will come to you more easily when you really need it.

Standing Up to the Thought Bullies

Your thoughts help frame your perception of a situation. It's one thing when a thought intends to be helpful and you make the mistake of pushing the panic button. But not all thoughts play nice. Some thoughts can be manipulative little bastards, just like that mean girl in high school who pretended to be your friend on the surface but secretly acted more like an enemy. Thought bullies can make you feel ashamed, worthless, bossed around, trapped, unlovable, alone, insecure, threatened, foolish, and ugly. And all too often, thought bullies stand directly between you and your goals.

What's the best way to handle a bully? Modern parenting experts would tell you that in order to bully-proof a child you need to empower her with strategies to handle the situation herself. Instead of shooting off an email to the school and insisting they punish the offending child, our kids benefit from knowing that we believe they are strong enough and smart enough to work things out. Now let's apply that same mindset to the **three types of self-defeating voices** that can linger with us into adulthood. You are strong enough and smart enough to stand up to the inner bullies who are sabotaging your happiness and well-being.

First is the *Ruthless Perfectionist*. She's a cross between Mommy Dearest and Martha Stewart, and her mission is to make you feel like the sludge on Bourbon Street the day after Mardi Gras. No matter what you do, it's not good enough. You will always be inadequate. You will never reach your goals. She hands out judgment like candy on Halloween and never misses an opportunity to be critical. "You're too ugly to be in the picture." "Don't you dare blow it by eating dessert." "You suck at your job." "You're such a lazy slob." "Look at those thighs—disgusting." This bully sets unrealistic standards and robs you of your ability to be compassionate toward yourself. Perfectionism is by far the most common and dangerous form of thought bullying. Listening to the ruthless perfectionist keeps you from living a life you want because she keeps you afraid, stuck in a tiny little jail cell, unable to make a move without fearing her wrath.

I love helping clients tame the next thought bully—the *Rebel Without a Cause*. Like a raging sixteen-year-old, full of angst, she'll turn on you in an instant and is guaranteed to fight you every step of the way, whatever your plans are. "You can't tell me what to do, MOM!" "Screw this crap; I'm running away." Your inner rebel hates structure and does not want to be controlled. She believes it's good to be bad and gets her power from coercing you to do the exact opposite of your intentions. When you set goals and don't follow through, you can thank your rebel voice, who doesn't want to deal with this behavior change BS. Her killer instinct is to label someone else as enemy number one and insist she is your only true friend. The rebel voice says to you, "Your boss is a jerk. Let's skip exercise, get cupcakes on the way home, and eat them in the car." This voice often shows up just as you begin to work on changing your habits, especially if you get tired or frustrated along the way. When you're putting energy into a new habit, she says "screw this shit" and "nobody's looking," but that is false. *You* are always there.

Spiral Up
EXPRESSIVE WRITING

How often do you spill your guts out like a thirteen-year-old girl to her diary? Pouring your thoughts onto a blank page helps you sift through emotions and see the experience from a different perspective. Often, when you commit to expressive writing exercises, you'll uncover stuff you didn't realize was there. This process also moves the information into a different storage center in your brain, which can decrease the intensity of feelings and help you work through difficulty with body kindness.

Get It Out There

You can't begin to fix what you don't know. Thoughts and feelings need a language:

- Writing lets you observe yourself. Think awareness, not judgment.

- Just get it on paper. Start writing, and don't worry if it's not well-written.

- Observe yourself like a scientist observes a subject.

- Be curious and honest. Tap into your thoughts, feelings, body expressions, and reactions.

- Don't worry if your words could hurt people. This is your private work.

- Write for at least fifteen minutes or until you think you're done. Then, read it.

When you try to understand the purpose of thoughts and feelings:

- It lowers anxiety and rumination on unhelpful, judgmental thoughts.

- You can begin to identify the root of a problem. You may see how much your response makes sense, given a situation. Or you may discover that you made mistakes.

- Taking this sacred "pause" makes room for feelings to pass naturally, without self-sabotage.

Actions: Can you think of one to three possible steps from here? Brené Brown reminds us, "When we own the story, we can write a brave new ending."

Write your ending and don't forget your humanness.

- I feel things.

- I make mistakes.

- It will be OK.

- I don't have to avoid pain.

- I can learn, grow, and improve my response next time.

What will you do for yourself in light of this emotional experience?

The *Tired Toddler.* Everyone has an inner child. Sometimes that child is a sniveling little whiney-pants like Veruca Salt in *Charlie and the Chocolate Factory*—"I want an Oompa Loompa now!" Kids haven't yet developed the rational part of their brain that understands the value of boundaries and they have difficulty regulating their emotions—hence, the tantrums. As adults, we should know that you can't always have whatever you want, whenever you want. Imagine taking a child to the toy store for one toy and they want more. You say, "Not right now" and get hit with "But that's not fairrrr," followed by a dramatic collapse and full-body convulsions. You take a deep breath and explain, "Sometimes you have to make a choice. Pick one toy. It's OK to be sad that there were several others you wanted. There will be more toys in the future."

Now imagine what the "toy" may represent for you: a second piece of cake, a marathon movie session at three a.m., or lingering in your pj's instead of rolling out of bed and into your workout clothes. Your child voice might say, "I don't want to get out of bed to exercise." "I want more ice cream now." "It's so hard to do the grocery shopping." "I hate cooking." It's one thing to make a conscious, calm decision that you want to enjoy a decadent dessert, but moderation will keep you from a toddler tummy ache. Own up to disliking food shopping and preparation, but do it anyway because you know it's important. You might be getting played by your inner child if she lets you avoid doing things you need to do because she whines, "I just don't wanna." The best way to end a tantrum is to blatantly ignore it and go about your day as planned—do your best to navigate around the raging toddler in aisle three and then hang out in the fresh produce department until you both calm down. When you're thinking "want" or "don't want," ask yourself, "What do I *need*?" to engage your adult-sounding, inner caregiver voice.

Beat a Thought Bully: Kill 'Em with Kindness

Hard as you may try, you can't force a thought bully to stop, but you don't have to let them control your life. What if you saw your thoughts as nothing more than stories that your mind is telling you? **You are not your thoughts. Thoughts have power only when you give it to them.** Thoughts are just the brain's way of filtering information, and just because you have a thought doesn't mean you have to act on it. What if you had the power to acknowledge an unhelpful thought without allowing it to take control of your next choice? You can do this by saying "hello" to your thought bully and then doing what any smart girl on the playground would do: You look the bully in the eye and then turn your back and go play with your real friends—your emotions.

The trick is to make room for all your feelings, even the bad ones. Think of each feeling as your temporary houseguest. Put on your hospitality pants and let that feeling know how much you appreciate its presence. Break out the good linens, the fine china, and the nice bottle of wine. Be grateful that emotion showed up, because it's communicating something important and it gives you a chance to practice your body kindness skills.

Imagine if your thought said, "Today sucked. Let's order pizza and eat it in bed," and instead of isolating yourself at home, you stopped at your favorite Thai restaurant and enjoyed a nice, calm, quiet dinner for one. Or what if your brain says, "Where's the wine? I can't handle these kids without it," and instead of reaching for the corkscrew you take a deep breath, allow the thought to pass, and decide to drink a tall glass of water. Or "I don't have the energy to work out. The boss was such a jerk," but you proceed to peacefully put on your exercise gear and dedicate a kickboxing session to proving your resilience.

When pain, fear, and uncertainty show up, throw a party and invite them to watch from the sidelines as you do a spontaneous body kindness freedom dance. That is how you can kick a nasty thought's nasty butt. I once had a client tell me, "Nobody is meaner to me than me. Frankly, if I was married to me, I'd divorce myself." The way you talk to yourself is a window into how you see yourself—and for many clients, changing their inner dialogue is one of the hardest steps in embracing a new way of life.

Don't be surprised if you try some of these techniques and start to see an immediate change in your thoughts. **Clients will often tell me that in as little as a few days they noticed a night-and-day difference in how they talk to themselves, including less frequent thought bullies, better strength in handling negative thoughts, and recognizing when their thoughts are actually trying to help, but they feel the urge to push the "panic button."** As time goes on you will continue to notice a difference, because you will have created a new way of appreciating negative emotions and tolerating unhelpful thoughts. I can't say they go away forever, but their power over you diminishes. Even I still catch myself in the occasional act of emotional eating or instinctually pinching a skin roll in the mirror once in a while. I like to think of my inner bully as the creepy character Malachai from Stephen King's *Children of the Corn*. When Malachai comes at me with an insult—"Look at that. Ya big blubber!"—I greet him coldly: "Hello Malachai." Then I do something uplifting to soothe my hurt feelings—like hug my kids for no reason. If that doesn't work, I try something else, knowing that as soon as I feel a little better, I win and Malachai loses.

What "name" can you give to your worst thought bullies? When your unhelpful thoughts take on a different persona, you will remember they aren't the *real* you and it's easier to stick up for yourself.

When How You Feel Impacts What You Want to Eat

Emotional eating is the act of eating food that has nothing to do with your need for nourishment. Typically, this occurs in response to stress or negative emotions, but it can also be triggered by positive feelings. Learning the different feelings of physical hunger and emotional hunger is a necessary step in overcoming emotional eating. Physical hunger is the biological signal that you need food. It is quite reliable, cued by an intricate dance of hormone signals, and tends to occur every three to five hours, depending on how much energy you burn and how much food you eat at a meal. Emotional "hunger" is triggered by some kind of event or experience that influences how you feel, independent of the time since your last meal, and may result in cravings for a specific type of food. You may not even know what it is, because you haven't really tuned in to what's going on. You just happen to be eating Nutella out of the jar at ten thirty at night in the dark. C'mon! I know I'm not the only one!

I'm not a betting woman, but if I were, I would double down on the statement "emotional eating impacts everyone." To some extent, we all make food choices that are impacted by our feelings, whether we're aware it's happening or not. Some people experience appetite loss when feeling stressed; others double up on carbs after a bad day. Any time you eat when you're not hungry, it's emotional eating—but not all emotional eating is a bad thing. It's possible to make a conscious choice to eat your feelings in calm, comfortable ways.

Your body kindness challenge is to get curious about what makes you reach for food and start to ask yourself what you are feeling. Even an emotion as benign as boredom can lead to emotional eating. Some major differentiators are how much you eat, how often, and the level of guilt or shame that follows those eating events. It's also important to remember that food cravings aren't always a result of biological hunger or your interest in enjoying a food you love. When you're stressed, cortisol is released, which triggers a desire for serotonin to calm you down. Serotonin is released when you eat foods rich in carbohydrates—hence the term "comfort foods." You might experience it as a craving you can't control, like someone else is driving the bus, and even if you hear yourself say, "Stop! No! Wait! Don't!" it feels like you can't. That's an impulse. When you repeatedly eat in response to feelings, it can become a habit. Then the next time you experience intense emotions, it might seem like your body is telling you to eat (it's usually something specific and probably not carrot sticks).

The good thing is that you're trying to connect and respond to your body's needs. Is it body kindness? Yes and no. Your body is saying "I need your attention," not necessarily "I need food." While eating can help you feel calm, it depends on how you eat (mindfully, with pleasure) and how much (comfortably full or too full after?) and whether you stay checked in with your emotions to fully enjoy the nourishment, even if you weren't that hungry. If you feel guilt, shame, and blame after eating, it's a downward spiral and it's not body kindness. If you are triggered to soothe, cope, or escape into negative choices, then it's time to ask yourself the universal body kindness question: *Is this helping to create a better life for myself?* Go through the mindfulness exercises from this chapter, like PACT (page 114) and the feelings sentence. Visualize the

emotional storm and surf past the urge to eat another bowl of cereal in bed. Your body is trying to connect with you, so show it some love by slowing down and thinking about your options to care for it.

Through over a decade of behavioral counseling, nearly everyone I have seen had a deeply conflicted relationship with food and admitted to emotional eating on some level. While the occasional boredom-driven chips and salsa in front of the tube won't cause long-term damage, many people struggle regularly and significantly with emotional eating. It can have a dramatic negative impact on your physical and emotional health and may even indicate an eating disorder.

You can break free from emotional eating if you are ready. It is a learned habit that can be unlearned with practice. All it requires is your commitment to pay attention to your body's signals and behaviors. It goes like this: There's a trigger, some kind of event or experience that influences how you feel. You get into a fight and you're mad and hurt—as you should be. The argument may have been a normal part of life, and your anger and sadness an inevitable and logical outcome after a fight. The problem really begins when there is a lack of self-awareness as to what happened and how it made you feel. You may be on automatic pilot, walking toward the fridge, and not even realize the inner dialogue has already started—"That wasn't sweet; let's eat sweets" or "I don't want to feel this pain; let's numb out with some pizza." The feelings are always there, but you may not even realize when a situation or emotion triggers a food craving. That's why the first step in PACT is *presence* and HALT (see below), another word for *pause*, reminds us of the power of calm, rational thinking. Your mindful observation will help you take care of yourself.

Body kindness activities can help you make good use of the energy that stressful moments bring. One of my go-tos is organizing. It's great for people who struggle with emotional eating or ruminating on bad thoughts because it occupies both your hands and your mind. Rather than think about how much you want to tear into a bag of chips,

Spiral Up

HALT—DO I NEED NOURISHMENT?

Before you reach for that cinnamon roll, check in on how you feel. Roll through a short list of emotions with the acronym HALT.

Hungry? Yep, you need to eat.

Angry, Lonely, or Tired (or any other emotion that is *not* hunger)? Nope, don't need to eat.

From here you can explore your triggers with the feelings sentence or move on to PACT to get to your next body kindness decision. For some, having the awareness that food won't solve their problems is enough of a reminder to bust out of the cycle and go do something—*anything*—besides eat.

Make a top ten list of things you can do when you feel intense emotions pulling you to the refrigerator. Your ideas should be easy, enjoyable, and soothing. Think of what could feel like a gentle hug—dancing to a song you love, sipping warm herbal tea, or lying flat on your back or taking your legs up the wall. Include more active, productive things you could always do, like give yourself a manicure or pedicure, organize papers lying around the house, or cross an item off your to-do list. Sometimes there's nothing more soothing than the sound of pen to paper making one swift line—done. The accomplishment you feel after completing one of these activities can be even more rewarding than the urge to "escape" your emotions with food.

HELP! I CAN'T STOP EMOTIONAL EATING!

If your emotions are intense, you may be experiencing a "hot state," in which your rational sense has gone on vacation.

RELAX

A centering activity will give you a chance to cool off. Try color breathing— imagine breathing in blue and green for calmness; and breathing out red to release stress.

DELAY

Take five minutes— or more. Rather than telling yourself, "Don't eat!" set a timer and defer the decision for 10 minutes. DING! Then use your calmer mind to reevaluate how you feel and what you want.

DISTRACT

While delaying, occupy your mind and hands with something that pleases you—Sudoku, jigsaw puzzles, gardening, a quick walk, even brushing your teeth—mint helps cut cravings.

THINK

If you're still craving a particular food, try putting these questions on index cards and ask yourself—this time and any other time you might be emotionally eating—"How much will I need to feel satisfied?" "How will I feel after eating it?" "Can I enjoy it calmly?"

Emotional eating is within your ability to identify and overcome!

focus your attention on making sense of your spice cabinet, or collecting and sorting the different stacks of stuff from around the house until your brain can't keep up with both thoughts. Beyond a distraction, organizing provides the benefits of a tangible outcome—a tidier, calmer space. Habits like these also give you a quick boost of endorphins from the satisfaction of seeing positive

BODY KINDNESS REFLECTION: Open up your journal to reflect on emotions. Are you trying too hard to control what you think and feel? For example, do you overeat, drink, or avoid exercise (or overexercise) to push away feelings or help you get through "bad" emotions? Name the different things you have done to try to deal with your emotions. For each activity, ask yourself, "Has this made life better or worse?" Describe how you know, with examples. Are you noticing downward spirals or upward spirals?

How can the mindfulness tools you've learned in this chapter help you handle intense thoughts and emotions in a body kindness way? Make note cards of your favorite tools. Place PACT, HALT, and the feelings sentence in places that will remind you to get in touch with what's happening, to allow whatever is there to be there, and then to choose an action that serves to make your life better.

results. When I see a client making poor use of energy to cope with stress, such as drinking alcohol, I'll jokingly say, "So how much do you have to drink in order for that work project to get done?" After we share a laugh, we can get down to planning rational responses to stressful situations. There is always a reason for emotions, but we don't always need to react to them. When bad things happen is often when we need body kindness the most. It's not the easiest time to be good to ourselves, but when we try, we grow stronger, spiraling up with every self-care choice, until we reach the calm after the emotional storm.

"Have a sense of gratitude to everything, even difficult emotions, because of their potential to wake you up."

—Pema Chödrön

Chapter 6

Make Room for More Fun

....

Feel Better, Do Better

Philosophy

Fun is like a body kindness vitamin you take to boost your mood and lift your spirit. The ability to let go and embrace the playful, silly side of life should be right up there with healthful food, sleep, and exercise on your self-care checklist. When you understand that your mental health is just as important as your physical health, fun no longer feels frivolous. Fun and laughter make our lives more meaningful and provide immeasurable long-term physical and mental health benefits. From improving your immune system to better memory and sleep habits, fun and laughter are powerful upward-spiral inducers that result in decreased stress and improved self-esteem.

BODY KINDNESS PILLARS
Having Fun Is Being Good to Yourself

LOVE: Filling your life with meaningful moments gives you joy in the present and for the future—in the form of memories you can cherish through the years.

CONNECT: Sense when your mind and body need a break from productivity to do something fun.

CARE: Pause to notice the fun you're having in life's big and little moments. Giving yourself the time you need to create joy is an essential part of self-care.

Find Your Fun Again

Whether it's being immersed in a hobby, finding the humor in a silly mishap, or noticing the joy in daily activities, every ounce of pleasure you can incorporate into life is worth pursuing. As adults, we spend so much time and energy focused on productivity and time management; do we know how to recognize fun when we see it? I am convinced that most people these days just aren't having enough fun. Don't get me wrong. Fun is there, but it practically has to scream its head off at you. "Hey! You! *Fun* here. Look at that awesome opportunity for us to get together. Whaddya say?" (silence) "Hellllooo? Is anybody home? Ugh, never mind." We have become so task-oriented in our daily lives that our thoughts constantly buzz about the next thing we have to do or the thing that happened yesterday that we can't let go of and we just forget to be here, now.

Noticing the fun in your everyday life is a form of mindfulness. A brief pause, just a few seconds of your time, is all it takes to connect with the present moment and observe how you feel. When you savor the good, you spiral up in energy and emotion, boost your happiness, and learn that what you're doing matters to you. I think of this as "little fun" because it's practically effortless and easily accessible to you every day.

Body kindness emphasizes seeking out an abundance of pleasure, not just

Spiral Up

Complete the following sentence: "Fun is _____ ." Think of at least five scenarios that are surefire smile-makers for you. Maybe it's "sipping hot cocoa by the fire with my family," "building blanket forts with the kids," or "shopping all day with my BFF." One of my personal favorites is "any time my toes are in water." How do you feel when you're having fun? What's one fun thing you want to do but have been putting off?

in day-to-day life but also on a larger scale. Plan for "big fun"—unstructured, unplugged playtime, whether it's engaging in a hobby you love on a regular basis or finally saying, "You know what, I have been talking about a trip to Europe for a decade, but I've never actually done it. The time is now!" Big fun requires more thought and effort and takes more of your time, but it pays off in happiness rewards and gratitude for all the gifts that make your life meaningful. If the practice of body kindness is about making self-care choices that create a better life, then *fun* is you living

that life right now. Not twenty pounds from now. Not once you've fixed your problems. *NOW.*

If you're stuck in the midst of a fun famine, it's time to find your way back to the land of plenty. All you need to do is say *"yes" to fun.* Believe that fun matters and make it happen in your own way, when you can. Usually when people wake up to the notion that fun is lacking in their life, time scarcity is to blame. There are two ways you can tackle a time dilemma—notice the good now (little fun) and make room for more good things in your life (big fun).

"Little Fun" Can Give Meaning to the Mundane

When someone tells me they are bored, lonely, or have a dull life, I ask them to describe their typical day. When you view things as a hassle, you can't feel the fun, and then what you're doing loses its

Are You in a Fun Famine?

* *

Fun Famine (*noun*): scarcity of laughter, silliness, and joy; the state of taking life too seriously; extreme absence of pleasure, as evidenced by severe facial expressions, bodily grunts, growls, and sighs, and the presence of a never-ending to-do list.

meaning. I'm not gleefully dancing my way into the grocery store every week, but if I were to complain about what a hassle it is, I can guarantee I won't have a good time. When your thoughts go down the path of pessimism—"What a drag! The lines! This sucks!"—you are truly missing an opportunity to appreciate the purpose of the present moment. Don't feign positivity. Just remember the value of your thoughts and actions.

Even grocery shopping has meaning to me. It makes eating well easier, cooking more convenient, and saves money—all things I care about. I think of it as a gift to myself so that I don't have to experience the negative consequences of an empty fridge or a frantic, last-minute call for delivery. When I get my reusable bags and strap my daughter in her car seat, I'm not just going grocery shopping. I'm going on a treasure hunt. I look for at least one fruit or vegetable I don't normally buy. I get excited about the possibility of discovering a new recipe or some other food trick that will make my life easier. Sometimes I challenge myself

to see how quickly I can get in and out of there by sticking to my list. I assign my daughter to help me spot items on the shelf. It gives us a chance to talk about food and build a positive connection to eating, which is very meaningful to me. And I never pass up the chance to peruse the 50-percent-off shelf of dented cans and other store deals. I am genuinely curious whether there is going to be anything that interests me. It's like the anticipation of garage sale bargain-hunting, and I might find a diamond in the rough! Laugh all you want, but I have saved a boatload of cash on wrapping paper, cards, kitchen gadgets, scented candles, and food. I don't automatically think of these benefits when I'm up too early on a Saturday fumbling through the kitchen trying to make my grocery list. But when my thoughts go spiraling down, I remind myself why I need to do this trip, and I remain committed to making the most of it.

Look for "little fun" in activities you do frequently and open yourself up to some surprises. A long, daunting car drive is an opportunity to listen to an audiobook that turns out to be decidedly pleasurable. Instead of just racing to get dinner on the table, think of meal prep as a calming reprieve from the busyness of your day job. Taking the dog to do his business can turn into a jaunt around the neighborhood—a pause that benefits both of you.

Your wandering mind will always take you somewhere else—into your phone, worrying about a work deadline, or checking items off a mental to-do list—but the activities that make up your day are often just one positive choice away from an upward spiral. Whenever possible, take a deep breath and try to move more slowly through your agenda. Use this gentle pause to savor the good that's happening in this moment. With a subtle shift in focus and perspective you'll see there really are many good moments to be had in your life. If this feels like a lot of gratitude, you're right! Appreciation sparks feelings of joy and contentment. It might not be your real idea of the best fun you can have, but this routine will pay off if you stick with it.

Finding Zen in the Kitchen

I have a confession. I don't enjoy cooking all the time. Some people love cooking. They would rather be in the kitchen than on a massage table, and I am not one of those people. My favorite part of cooking is the creativity. I love discovering a new simple, quick, and delicious way to enjoy eating. But when it comes to the grind of getting dinner on the table by 6:00, "fun" is not the first word that comes to mind. One of the things that has really helped me and a few of my kitchen-phobic friends is a commitment to changing our attitudes and making food preparation a mindful experience—and it works. All you do is find little ways of being in the moment and letting go. Just like relaxing a sore muscle, you breathe into the discomfort and find your relief.

Combining cooking and meditation is a life-enhancing experience for your mind and body. In fact, Buddhist monks are convinced that the mood in the kitchen even affects the health and digestion of food. When you take the time to pay attention to the sights, sounds, and smells of your food and the environment around you, it slows down the process and can make mealtime more of a gift than a chore.

You can apply this Zen-inspired mindset to other areas of health and wellness—from fitness to sleep to sex. Paying attention brings you the gift of presence.

ZEN IN THE KITCHEN

COOKING AND MEDITATION BLEND BEAUTIFULLY

Combine cooking and meditation for an enhancing experience!

Benefits

Increase creativity, alleviate depression, better mood, less stress, improvements to mindful eating, and more satisfying meals

Zen up with a few long, slow, deep breaths.

Push play on some calm instrumental music or ambient sound-track—like rainfall, ocean, or forest sounds.

Grab your recipe, ingredients, and get ready to go—slow.

USE ALL OF YOUR SENSES

SIGHT
Take a look at the beautiful colors while you're cooking.

TASTE
Chefs always taste their food as they cook. Go for it. What do you notice?

AROMA
As your food cooks, notice how the aroma changes. What pleasant aromas do you notice?

SOUND
From chopping to sizzling, notice the various sounds of cooking.

BONUS! MENTAL CLARITY
Being precise when measuring ingredients enhances focus.

Discover the Fun in Fitness

Finding the crossroads between self-care and joyful living is at the heart of everything I teach my clients. For me, this journey blossomed several years ago when I discovered yoga. Before my body kindness "awakening," I had always been the one at the gym wearing my "No Pain, No Gain" tank top. **For most of my adult life, I'd headed straight for the cardio machines, which I nicknamed the Dreadmill and the Swearmaster. It felt normal to hate exercise.** I was going to do it, but I wasn't going to like it. Exercise was "hard."

I didn't realize how disempowering this mindset was for me until I wandered into my first yoga class. For several weeks I walked past an "Opening Soon" sign for a yoga studio during my daily latte fix at Starbucks in downtown DC, and my curiosity was piqued. I happened to be wearing workout gear when the sign changed to read "Grand Opening Today." So with a borrowed yoga mat and no preconceived ideas, I settled into my first downward-facing dog and was instantly hooked. From that moment on, I began to realize that exercise had beneficial purpose beyond calorie burns. There was so much to learn, from the terminology and names of poses to the mindset of non-judgment and self-compassion. Yoga even taught me how to breathe correctly, and use my breath to regulate my mood. Yoga was challenging, but it wasn't "hard." I wanted to be there. I wanted to learn and grow. I believed I could rise to the challenges yoga presented me. I could experience the discomfort of a pose without judging myself.

Perhaps most important, I was enjoying myself and working out at the same time, and now I apply this yoga mindset to all forms of exercise. Whether I'm running in the park or trying to keep my balance in a solidcore class, I know that I can enjoy all types of exercise and challenge myself when the focus is on how I feel in the moment instead of getting a tighter tush. Exercise is also an opportunity to unleash your playful side. Would you try a ballroom dancing or belly dancing class? Would you hop in a canoe and paddle down the river? When you enjoy yourself during exercise, you'll be more consistent with it, and you'll reap the rewards.

Spiral Up
A FUN REFLECTION

Think about how you have spent the last few days. Did you have some fun? Do you naturally pause to notice the good time you're already having? Can you think of any activities you do regularly that could use a mindset shift? What can you do to go from a "little fun" famine to feast? Get out that journal and start planning more fun in your life!

Laughing for Fun's Sake

Why do people love memes and emojis on social media? Because we're all dying to laugh a little. A chuckle from a silly riddle (When is it the best time to go to the dentist? *Tooth hurty.*) and boisterous laughter from a night of Cards Against Humanity is like medicine for a bad mood. When you laugh, your brain floods with dopamine and serotonin, and the stress hormones cortisol and epinephrine drop, helping you to relax. Laughter is a natural "chill pill" and health enhancer. It supports memory, improves sleep quality, helps fight depression and anxiety, and bolsters the immune system. It also helps prevent heart attacks, boosts creativity, relieves muscle tension, improves blood flow and increases oxygen throughout the body, and raises pain tolerance. Also, believe it or not, laughter is a form of exercise. Vigorous laughter increases the heart rate, deepens breathing, and engages muscles in the face, stomach, and diaphragm. Have you ever laughed so hard it felt like you did a hundred sit-ups? I sure hope so.

Maybe laughter can't replace chemotherapy or antibiotics, but its healing powers are no joke. Laughter is vital to good health, and I'm convinced it's more important for long-term well-being than any lab result or number you see on a scale. A simple commitment to laugh more often can lead to long-term improvements in your mood, which will naturally support your other body kindness goals. Once you start paying attention to how often you laugh (or the opposite), it becomes easier to choose lightheartedness more often, and this can positively affect your whole outlook on life. Like the day I overflowed an entire pot of coffee only to turn around and find my daughter pouring a container of orange juice down the kitchen cabinets. My quick decision to laugh hysterically at our mutual mess was the only thing that got us both out the door in one piece that morning!

To laugh more is one of those idealistic thoughts we have when dreaming about what a good life looks like. We want to live in the moment, love like there's no tomorrow, and laugh every day. Of all life's desires, I can't think of many things more accessible than laughter as a gateway to upward spirals of fun. Let's unleash laughter in all its wonderful forms. Let's giggle, crack up, and roar with intention. Next time you laugh, pause for a second and notice—what tickled your funny bone, who was with you to enjoy it, and how do you feel in body and mind when you're laughing? The best laughter unexpectedly sneaks into your ordinary life. Maybe it's there to remind you that having fun is good for you.

Growing "Big Fun"

Does it always feel like there's something more important you should be doing? What if having fun was at the top of the list? Learning to make time for "big fun"—things you do on purpose for enjoyment—will help you be more effective, efficient, energetic, confident, and creative in the long run. But like any other body kindness practice, fun has to be done consistently in order to become a habit. Many people simply do not make personal enjoyment and leisure a priority. It's one thing to *know* that you should take care of yourself so you can take care of others, but another to commit time, money, and resources to put fun on your body kindness to-do list. If you're having a hard time going from thinking about fun to making it happen, ask yourself "Why?" Is there a part of you that thinks you don't deserve to have fun? What is more important than your own well-being? How can you possibly keep up all these important things if you don't recharge your own battery? Creating big fun in your life starts with small efforts and grows from there.

We often call taking a break "downtime," but I think it's more appropriate to call it "uptime" because it spirals you up, lifts your mood, and energizes you. One small thing you can do is start giving yourself little chunks of time to replenish and uplift. I call these precious moments *Happy Hours* (no drinking required). Happy Hours help you feel good now and in the future. They heighten your confidence that you are taking care of yourself as you surf the waves of life (sometimes wiping out and falling flat on your ass). You can get started with Happy Hours right now by taking a few minutes—or seconds—out of your day to check in with yourself and boost your well-being with anything that helps you feel good. Do you need a drink of water? A quick stretch? Some music while you read or work? You can do a Happy Hour for any length of time—take the day if you can!

We all have the power to grow positive emotions and become happier, healthier, and more satisfied. Even a very depressed person can increase happiness by making one small, positive choice at a time. Think for a minute: If you had an extra hour or two that you could use only for genuine fun, what would you do? Dream big! Because when your life and your calendar are full of things to look forward to, you are less likely to seek out false pleasures to soothe away bad feelings. What you do for your big fun brings meaning and purpose into your life, and makes lasting, positive change possible.

It's still amazing to me when I think about helping people reach their health-related goals just by telling them to go out and have a good time! While it seems simple enough to do, time and again I've watched clients struggle to find more joy in their busy lives. The busier you feel (I'm talking to you—parents, perfectionists, and people-pleasers), the more likely you are to sit there with arms crossed, refusing to do anything nice for yourself. I get it. My arms are crossed, too. We're busy, tired, overwhelmed, and don't want to waste precious brain cells deciding what to do for fun, not to mention taking on the work to plan it all. Why shouldn't there be more fun in our lives? Don't limit yourself to things you already know you enjoy. There are added physical and mental benefits from being open to new experiences.

Feeling the Flow

One essential element of a happy, meaningful life is the ability to get lost in experiences you find challenging, enjoyable, and rewarding. Hungarian psychologist Mihaly Csikszentmihalyi coined the term "flow state" to describe the experience of being so absorbed with concentration in one activity that you lose track of time and nothing else seems to matter. His lifelong study of happiness psychology led to the discovery that people are happiest when they are in a flow state, aka "in the zone" or "in the groove." So it stands to reason that making time for these types of activities in our lives is an important part of self-care. What areas and activities come to mind when you think about flow state? Chess players, musicians, artists, and athletes have all been studied to verify the power of this psychological phenomenon. Thankfully, you don't have to be an expert at something to get lost in enjoyment. There's a reason adult coloring books have exploded in popularity. From intricate mandalas to flowery swear words, if you can hold a crayon, you can get lost in the feel-good flow state.

Listening to music is an activity where almost anyone can escape or get inspired, encouraged, or motivated—sometimes all in one song. Whether you're a fan of Mozart or Metallica, the therapeutic benefits of music have been celebrated and researched for centuries. Music has been dubbed a natural antidepressant for its ability to change your outlook and disposition, altering it for hours or even days.

Anything fun that puts you in a flow state can be healthy for you. If you get pleasure out of baking, gifting, and sharing desserts (including enjoying them yourself), then you are lifting your spirits and your mood and connecting with others. It makes you happier and adds to your energy, and from that foundation you're in a great place for other body kindness choices.

Have you ever taken a mental health day and played hooky from it all? When I start daydreaming about this—and I do!—it usually means it's time to stop what I'm doing and find something fun to do, even just for a moment. My friend Pleasance Silicki, a professional yoga instructor in Washington, DC, swears that the key to her success in business and in helping others comes from her frequent recalibration retreats. By spending a day in silence or flying off to someplace amazing for a week of yoga and meditation—she practices what she preaches, and I swear the positive energy radiates from her. Talk about body kindness. You don't have to have a passport just to reboot yourself, but why not take a day for some big fun?

Entertaining with Joy

I'm a social butterfly and love to show people a good time. For me, hosting parties offers a chance for great big fun. I get to catch up with people, laugh with them, and exchange stories over good food and drink. I seem to spiral

Spiral Up
FIND YOUR FUN

⏺ ⏺

Grab your journal. Match the first activities that come to your mind with these signs of a genuinely fun experience.

* You're smiling (inside or out).

* You can't wait to do it again.

* You don't want it to end.

* You lose track of time.

* You feel good afterward.

* Spontaneous laughter erupts!

* Your spirit feels lighter.

* Your worries disappear.

When was the last time you participated in these activities? What are ways you can enjoy them more often and more fully? Include things you find enjoyable in daily life and commit to savoring the fun a little more in these moments.

up all night long. But you know how the idea of throwing a big party sounds better than the reality of all the work involved in pulling it off? In my head, the parties I plan are amazing. But it never fails—the day before the big event I'm overwhelmed and dreading it. Every other word out of my mouth is an expletive and I have one finger poised to hit send on my drafted email canceling the party due to an "unexpected illness." But when I remind myself of all the shared joy that getting together brings people—and realize these events aren't about having the perfect plan—I take a deep breath and bust into get-it-done mode. I've learned sometimes you have to go through a little muck to get to good fun. Planning can be more joyful, too, when you focus on the mood you want your gathering to bring. My menu planning with joy "cheat sheet" helps you think through the big decisions that come with planning a menu for your special guests.

MENU PLANNING WITH JOY

Overcome dinner dread by thinking with your heart.

Desire: Do you want to impress or comfort? Do you want to make food the focus or have simple nourishment with quick cleanup while you connect with your guests? Make the meal a star or a cameo appearance.

Desires

Guests

Season

Available resources

Function

Weather

Cravings

Occasion

Function:
For cheering up a friend, make her favorite dish or Google "mood boosting foods." Want to up your kids' vitamin intake? Go for veggies tucked inside a savory casserole. Or make a grilled fruit dessert.

Occasion:
Colorful and fun for a celebration! Full of heart and soul for a consolation. A special presentation for a happy memory.

Cravings:
Are there foods you'd like to taste, crunch, try out, or revisit?

Season:
Seasonal ingredients contribute to a meal's freshness, color, and taste. Fresh corn and tomatoes eaten outdoors. Roasted root vegetables eaten by the fire.

Available Resources:
Think about time, money, and what's in the cabinet. There can be as much love and elegance in pasta and sauce as in a more elaborate recipe.

Weather:
Dining al fresco always feels fun and can eliminate the need to clean house! Pack up a basket and head to the local park.

Guests:
What preferences or needs do your guests have?

Desperately Seeking Smiles

There is no one size fits all approach to fun. It's anything you want it to be. It's alone time. Family time. Game time. Girl time. It's drinking homemade margaritas on your patio in the mid-afternoon or running through the sprinkler with your kids. It's detaching from work for the entire weekend to invest in the rest of your life. Fun means finally stopping at that roadside stand or quirky little antique store you've driven by for years. It's realizing that you deserve to make time for your workout *and* hang out with a friend, instead of always choosing the more productive option.

Please don't wait for permission to embrace silliness and joy. No one is going to give it to you, and there is a lot to be gained from letting your guard down and risking vulnerability. A friend recently told me about a party she attended with a live band. She loved the music but felt "too cool and too cranky" to do anything more than just tap her foot and sway her hips like a wallflower. Eventually more and more people made their way to the dance floor, and she was slowly getting outnumbered on the sidelines. When she finally decided to let go and get down with the rest of them, not only did she have fun—she pushed a personal boundary. Each time we do this, life repays us tenfold with opportunities to do it again. Be open to the idea of trying something fun, new, and exciting.

Spontaneous joy can sneak up and delight you, bringing you a new experience, teaching you something, and helping you learn and grow. But this isn't something you can schedule into the calendar—all you need is an open heart and mind. The best way to ask life for more fun is by seeking out new experiences. Start by saying "yes" more often, especially when you're feeling curious but a little fearful at the same time! Be open to adventure! When you notice a food that looks good on another person's plate—ask the waiter to give you "what they're having." Or maybe you've planned an afternoon of shopping and chores, but someone offers you tickets to a show or sporting event. Time for a change of plans!

You be you. Just don't let a fear of fun make your body kindness practice more difficult than it needs to be, and consult your inner happiness meter as often as possible. Ask yourself, "What would make me feel content, peaceful, or joyful right now?" This can apply to food choices and exercise. Better yet, the next time you start to reach for a glass of wine or a cupcake after a long day, go do something fun for thirty minutes and then rethink your choice. Go ahead and have the drink or dessert if you really want it—just make sure you are mindfully savoring the experience and not trying to cover up dullness. You'll find that bringing fun back into your life will warm your heart and fill your mind with sweet memories.

BODY KINDNESS REFLECTION: Spend fifteen minutes planning some good, honest fun in your life. What are your Happy Hours? Make a list of interests and hobbies that are calling your name. Write down what you would do if you didn't have responsibilities tomorrow and then brainstorm what it would take to make it happen. Chances are, you'll have fun just making plans. Now take one step, no matter how small or insignificant—just one thing that makes you smile or puts you a step closer to something on that list!

"We didn't realize we were making memories, we just knew we were having fun."

—Unknown

Chapter 7

Bouncing Back and Growing Stronger

Body Kindness Enhances Resilience

Philosophy

Everyone experiences stress, sometimes big and sometimes small. High-intensity emotions over a period of time can make you feel like the solid ground is crumbling at your feet. Body kindness is most difficult when you feel unable to handle what's coming at you. Resilience, or the ability to bounce back from adversity, is a skill that some people seem to have naturally and anyone can build. Becoming stronger after negative life events, including significant traumas like losing a loved one, divorce, or losing a job, is called post-traumatic growth. You can strengthen your emotional fitness by cultivating skills to help you accept and reframe adversity as a natural part of life and a growth opportunity. This resilience will equip you to continue making body-kind decisions even during the most stressful situations.

BODY KINDNESS PILLARS
Bounce Back from Bad

LOVE: When you're at a low point, the love you have for yourself will ultimately nurture your healing process.

CONNECT: When you're in the middle of bouncing back, connection will help you find the real you again.

CARE: When you make body kindness choices, you mend your heart and mind, which helps you recover faster.

The Life-Enhancing Benefits of Stress

"I'm so stressed." When was the last time you said or thought that? You're not alone. The modern-day response to "How was your day?" has somehow become "Crazy." Stress impacts most Americans on a daily basis—in fact, it's killing us. According to the American Psychological Association's 2015 Stress in America survey, chronic stress is linked to six leading causes of death. And for those of us not dying from it, many are still experiencing unprecedented incidences of anxiety, depression, and insomnia from the frantic pace of life.

"Stress is bad." This is the message I was inundated with throughout my education, and I always believed that my own life experiences were more proof of the same. Overwhelming stress was the primary trigger that would send me diving face-first into a pint of ice cream, every single time. Early in my career I shared this stress-is-harmful mindset with everyone—family, friends, and clients. "It's overwhelming you, it leads to pain and suffering, and you need to avoid it at all costs." I was a full-fledged, card-carrying stress fearmonger. Unfortunately I was operating under a deep misconception about the nature of stress, and despite my best intentions to help people relieve stress, I was probably making things worse. Reinforcing the belief that my clients couldn't handle stress actually reduced their motivation to take action. **It's not the stress that hurts you, it's**

Spiral Up

Write in your journal about two bad experiences in your life, one big and one small. Describe what happened, how it made you feel, how it may have impacted your choices, your physical or mental health. Describe how you worked through it. Reflecting back, in which ways did you practice body kindness? How is it difficult to be good to yourself when bad things happen? How does it benefit you to practice body kindness when life knocks you down?

---

your fear that you don't have what it takes to make it through.

Stress is a natural physiological reaction to perceived danger. The body reacts immediately to stress with physical changes, and a cascade of hormones causes increases in heart rate, a flushed face, and a surge of energy. Next up is the behavioral response (ice cream or a deep breath?), and then what's left is our subjective experience (how we feel about what we just did). The response to stress is key. What do you do with the energy you get from stress?

Stanford University professor Kelly McGonigal's book *The Upside of Stress* helped me give myself permission to feel stress and authentically believe I was going to come out of it OK. McGonigal asserted that stress is your body's way of saying "this matters to me." By responding to a stressful situation with the thought "my body is responding to something I care about," I reduced the power fear had over me. In fact, I could make good use of the energy stress gave me by doing something helpful, like taking one huge massive deep breath in, holding it, then releasing it as slowly as I could, or going into downward-facing dog and letting out three of the loudest "lion's breaths" I could muster.

If we're not mindful of our challenges and how they make us feel, it can lead to bad choices that aren't in line with our desire to practice body kindness. No amount of food, alcohol, or punishing exercise takes away bad feelings, rights wrongdoings, or prevents unwanted events in life. If we don't take care of ourselves, we can fall into a deep downward spiral of negative emotions, bad choices, low energy, prolonged sadness, emotional distress, or depression. But the beautiful news is that no matter how big or small your setback, and no matter how you have handled stress in the past, you can build your skills to bounce back faster than ever and even become a stronger person.

How Big Is Your Stuff?

My uncle Paul gave me one of the best pieces of advice I've ever received. He said, "Beck, there's little stuff and big stuff. You need to decide what type of stuff you're in before you make decisions. Otherwise, you could wind up in a whole load of crap for no good reason." Accurately assessing the magnitude of the situation is a crucial skill because it can subdue unnecessary panic and unraveling emotions, which lead to bad choices. Ask yourself, "Will this matter in a year?" Many of the things we worry about don't even matter in a day. Your spouse made a hurtful joke or your coworker left a mess in the shared kitchen. Disappointments, mistakes, and misunderstandings are inevitable parts of life, and you get to decide how much you let this "little stuff" affect you.

A Story of Little Stuff

I was standing in the kitchen pouring a cup of coffee when my three-year-old, Audrey, cried out with a helpless-sounding "Mommy." Suddenly I had a flash vision—completely unrelated to where I was and what we were doing. I was on an airplane with my daughters and we were in rough turbulence. The plane was having problems. "What would I do if it were going down?" I thought. I imagined myself saying, "It's OK, Audrey. Hold Mommy's hand. Let's sing." Then I panicked. "What about my infant, Isla?" I quickly decided I'd nurse her to bring her comfort. My anxiety lifted briefly as I thought to myself, "Just be there for your kids." But my heart started racing again when I had another flash. As the plane was headed toward the earth, it broke apart and Isla flew out of my arms. My eyes welled with tears at the horrific thought of not being able to be there for my children when they needed me most, and I nearly began sobbing over Audrey's waffles. "STOP!" I yelled in my head. "STOP IT NOW. You are not on a crashing airplane. You are in your kitchen having breakfast with your daughter before preschool." I snapped out of it, but it was tough to shake my emotions. I felt heartbroken, distraught, and helpless all at once. I got curious. Why did my mind spin off like that? What's going on with me *for real*? It took all of two seconds for me to get it. I was feeling more intense stress than usual. I was on a book deadline, starting a podcast, finishing year-end business operations, and trying to get a family of four packed for a trip over the holidays. We were leaving the following day. The house was a mess and the suitcases sat empty next to a pile of laundry. My schedule was bouncing all over the place, which normally is fine, but not this time. I was under-sleeping and I hadn't made exercise a priority in a few days—two of my most important body kindness habits. But none of this "stuff"—the messy house, the trip, even the holiday preparations—none of it was going to matter in a year and none of it was worth losing health and happiness over. It was *all* little stuff. I was temporarily overwhelmed and nothing more. Everyone was OK. I had a momentary lapse in sanity and my mind wandered to dark places. That's all. I caught myself in the downward spiral. I worked my way through PACT, and instead of throwing my self-care goals out the window, I revisited them and found my way through the little stuff.

A Story of Big Stuff

"What happened last night?" Michelle sheepishly asked her husband when she woke up with a splitting headache, cotton mouth, and a bad case of the spinning rooms. "Well, let's see. You were hanging on George right in front of his girlfriend. You told everyone we haven't had sex in months. You started undressing while our neighbors were still over, so I took you up to bed. You puked on me on the way up the stairs." Michelle responded quietly, "Oh. I must have blacked out." "Are you surprised?"

he retorted. "It's like a regular thing with you. You're either an alcoholic or a loser." Michelle was silent. She got a glass of water, some Tylenol, and went back to bed while her husband took care of their two children most of the day. When she emerged later, sober, she decided she did not want her life to be like this, and contacted an intensive treatment program for alcohol abuse.

You don't just wake up one day and decide to go get therapy without having lots of "big stuff" happen. It wasn't just alcohol—Michelle had a history of an eating disorder, perfectionism, and low self-esteem, all intersecting and manifesting in various ways. Most of her life was full of little stuff and big stuff. Michelle knew one thing. Her "stuff" was not creating a better life. She took an action to help her deal with it all and work on becoming the person she truly wants to be. Through treatment, Michelle has learned that perfectionism and her harsh inner critic left her no room to be human. Her thoughts and feelings were so overwhelming—restricting food, over-exercising, and drinking to excess were all ways she exuded "fake control." She was trying to cope with stress, but she was taking the wrong approach. She was numbing. Somewhere along the way, she got buried beneath all the unrelenting negative thoughts and feelings that were controlling her life. Thankfully, Michelle is resilient. She was able to wake herself up from a long, tumultuous downward spiral and begin to spiral up, one choice

Spiral Up
WAYS TO BOUNCE BACK

When your feelings say, "Hey, something's not right," it can be uplifting to cut yourself some slack and give yourself a mini-break, a time-out, a pause.

* Take a minute—take an hour—or take a day.

* Have faith and practice it by praying or meditating.

* Walk the dog and observe the "little things": trees, flowers, dirt.

* Do something nice for someone.

* Read a book—it will help you think of a story different from yours.

* Get silly . . . Hula-Hoop, juggle, sing a song.

* Make a soothing cup of tea.

* Pet a furry creature.

* Listen to some reliably mood-lifting or soothing music.

* Breathe and find something to be grateful for.

* Lie down and rest or nap.

* Get yourself up and do some exercise to work the feelings out of your system.

* Bonus: Exercise outdoors where nature can bring joy faster.

* Talk about your feelings, cry, seek connection.

* Cross everything else off your to-do list—then do something that feels good.

* Recall a past triumph—you are resourceful.

* Try a new recipe, workout, or other interest.

* Surround yourself with love in a happy place.

FOR A WORKDAY REBOOT:

* Take recess at work with a jump rope or a piece of chalk and a hopscotch board.

* Keep a satchel of fun at your desk: bubbles, Play-Doh, knock-knock jokes, adult coloring books, mini Zen garden.

* Smile, fake it until you make it, and take a few silly selfies while laughing with (not at!) yourself.

* Reflect on three good things—in your life, that you've seen, that you can do, etc.

* Unleash your inner Buddha with deep breaths, loving-kindness meditation (Chapter 10), lavender oil, or a home spa treatment.

* Keep a "glory folder"—rereading congratulatory emails, thank-you cards, or any kind messages can reignite good feelings.

at a time. And now she is learning just how strong she truly is. During treatment, Michelle learned to accept herself, value her past, and look toward the future—the essential elements to overcoming life's big stuff.

....

Look for the Lesson

....

Little and big problems can cloud our focus on body kindness, even though taking care of ourselves fuels the energy and perspective we need to find our way through. There is an opportunity to learn and grow from every bad experience in life. Ask yourself these questions: "What's the lesson? How can this situation help me? What's the most optimistic point of view I can take here?" Can you express gratitude for the difficulty you're facing? Obviously, that is not going to work for all bad things. It's not easy to cultivate gratitude after the death of a loved one or the loss of a job. But you can re-create the story of your loss. Can you find meaning in it? Focus your energy on bouncing back by looking for the good again, in whatever way possible. Any time you allow yourself to think positively, your brain secretes more DHEA hormone, which helps you learn and grow, fostering your resilience. Feeling better and spiraling upward happens one choice at a time, one day at a time.

In my little stuff story, I could appreciate that my mental panic led me to acknowledge my real-life stress. I was grateful for the painful emotions I felt because they were appropriate to the disastrous scenario playing in my head. It told me my body and mind were working—sort of. What I did not do was wallow in negative emotions all day long. I could have allowed the day to downward spiral, from a hypercritical "you suck" dialogue to emotional eating, or running to bed and avoiding my to-do list. But I didn't do that. I found a lesson, hugged my daughter, and took a walk to my favorite bookstore and coffeehouse. I enjoyed a croissant as well as a glimpse of the newest releases. I bounced back by making one spiral-up choice at a time, and even after I took a little extra time for myself, the important things managed to get done, and we all made it to the plane on time, suitcases fully packed.

When big stuff happens, you aren't going to solve it by taking a walk or a bubble bath. Dealing with something big calls for the big guns: patience, compassion, flexibility, determination, hope, and an open mind. Big stuff takes time, but you willingly give it because you love yourself. Deep down you want a better life. Something you care about is at stake, and you are going to march on and deal with what comes at you. Body kindness jumps in at a vitally important time to keep you spiraling up in energy and mood, growing through your difficulty.

Someone else's big stuff can be yours, too, like a good friend of mine whose teenage daughter was dealing with depression. This family trauma put a dark, overwhelming cloud over my friend's body kindness abilities. But staying committed to a healthy life allowed her to acknowledge her own downward spirals, including the guilt-ridden "good mother" inside her head, telling her she couldn't make time to see her friends or exercise. And then she chose to do those things anyway because they matter. It's this "me first" mindset that helps her be who she needs to be for her daughter—a strong, loving mother who supports her as she kicks depression's sorry little you-know-what. **Think of the "lessons" of big stuff like strength training. It helps you practice your skills of self-care, handling emotions, and problem-solving with real, workable solutions.** Body kindness means taking your mental health seriously, understanding that the mind and body are connected, making time for meditation, and appreciating life's joys, just to name a few. Revisit the stories you journaled about at the start of the chapter. Think about the lessons and the most optimistic viewpoint you can take. Find examples of

Spiral Up
LITTLE STUFF AND BIG STUFF MATTER

For the little stuff: Are you an over-reactor? Do you treat your little stuff like big stuff? What little things have caused you to feel negative emotions and cope in unhelpful ways? Write about it in your journal. Think about the mindfulness tools you could use to identify what you want to do when you're experiencing the little "this won't matter in a year" stuff. Now reflect on the big stuff in your life, from the past or present. What skills did you gain from getting through that time? What's the lesson? How can you learn and grow? What examples of resilience do you have? How would you have liked to handle your big stuff?

your strength, growth opportunities, and resilience—even if you made mistakes handling the stress. There's no such thing as a stress-free life. Strive to become aware of your big stuff and little stuff when it's happening, and take actions you need to get through difficulty.

Let Good Enough Be Good Enough

When you are trying to bounce back, mindset is everything. Extreme, perfectionistic thinking is the stuff of downward spirals. Go for *progress, not perfection*. Being satisfied with "good enough" allows you to move on, save brainpower, and avoid overthinking, which can have a direct impact on your body kindness choices.

Many of us need to practice being imperfect and self-compassionate—because it doesn't always come easy. Within Michelle's first week of sobriety, she began to have more intense sugar cravings than ever before. Always striving to be the perfect eater, she felt guilty when she didn't eat well. But the sugar cravings felt overwhelming (and are a biological response to giving up alcohol when you've become addicted to it). Her food choices reflected a "total cop-out on health" in her mind—lots of sugary desserts, pasta, pancakes, takeout food, and nary a fruit or vegetable with most meals.

Frustrated and hoping to feel better, she decided to do a fruit and vegetable juice cleanse to restart healthful habits. But all she got was hunger pangs within hours and downright anger within a few days. When she told her doctor what she was doing and why, Michelle got the reprieve she needed. "Stop that right away," her doctor said, "and go eat the regular, healthful food you need." After talking more with her doctor and me, Michelle realized that giving up alcohol left her with a void in coping strategies. In a sense, food replaced drinking as a way to deal with life and she needed to allow for that at times. Michelle decided she would stop trying to be so perfect with food at this time in her life. "I need to stop judging myself. If it's pancakes and fruit for dinner, it's OK. If it's pasta, I can add mushrooms and tomato sauce. I don't have to make quinoa and kale salads for me and something else for the kids."

How to Bounce Back Big the Body Kindness Way

We all know people who have been through the wringer, and we've been those people too. We know bad events don't last forever. But if there's a way to help us treat ourselves better, why not do it? Here's my six-step plan for bouncing back with body kindness.

1 Commit to using body kindness as a guide for your bounce back. This is a crucial first step because you need a starting point and a point to return to in case you need to start over.

2 Feel your pain and give yourself permission to feel better. Allow your negative emotions to fully express themselves by validating and acknowledging them. You need to feel the pain, but you can also feel good again. People close to me have admitted they feel guilty about feeling good so close to a tragedy in their life. They think they should suppress good feelings for longer. Not true. Feeling bad is part of what leads to feeling good. You can be kind to yourself while you work through difficulty and make your life better at the same time.

3 Make room for a daily sacred pause. Whether you pray, meditate, repeat affirmations, journal, or do a little bit of everything, now is the time you need to consistently take these pauses to just be. Express your spirituality in whatever form(s) suit you and realize that your soul is a valuable part of this universe. Plan and schedule purposeful body kindness routines.

4 You've laid your bounce back foundation, so now taking action on body kindness should go a little more smoothly. There is tremendous comfort in routines, especially during the unreliable and difficult time of bounce backs. Follow a plan instead of making decisions. What you do for body kindness during a bounce back, like any other time, is up to you. Taking care of yourself through food,

Spiral Up
BOUNCE BACK BY
GROWING YOUR MIND

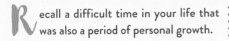

Recall a difficult time in your life that was also a period of personal growth.

* *What made this time* challenging or stressful for you?

* *What did you care* most about? What worries or concerns were present?

* *What did you do* to support yourself? How were you supported through this experience by others?

* *How did this experience* change how you viewed yourself, others, or life itself? What did you learn about yourself?

* *What is an example* of something you have you been able to do, face, or embrace since that time, that you are able to appreciate about yourself?

* *If you could go back in time* and give yourself some words of encouragement during that stressful period, what would you say?

---

fitness, fun, and sleep will heal your mind and body.

5 Forgive. You will make mistakes during your bounce back efforts and you'll need to forgive yourself. Or perhaps someone important to you will be insensitive, be hurtful, or commit another transgression and you'll feel knocked down. Forgive them. You need to be forgiving to keep moving forward. Your mental energy is better served toward your bounce back. Desmond Tutu says, "Without forgiveness, there's no future."

6 Wait for it. Indeed, practicing body kindness helps you bounce back faster, but you're not in a race. It's not like one day you're suffering and the next you're fine. Don't tell yourself you're failing when your bounce back takes longer than you want it to. Keep practicing body kindness through every step of the journey.

Getting Back to Good Again

The father of positive psychology, Martin Seligman, PhD, provides an acronym for happiness, which he defines as subjective well-being. This is not simply the fleeting state of happiness, but an overall assessment of your life having meaning and purpose, a long-term happiness.

Seligman's acronym, PERMA, has stood up to the rigor of decades of psychology research and has shown to be a valid way of measuring happiness. PERMA was an inspiration to me in aligning the body kindness philosophy with a positive state of well-being. PERMA can be particularly helpful during a bounce back because it reminds you what matters most in life.

P = POSITIVE EMOTIONS. Your ability to generate good feelings (spiral up!).

E = ENGAGEMENT. That feeling when your enjoyment and interest are pure—whether you're working, parenting, socializing, or engaged in a hobby (fun!).

R = RELATIONSHIPS. Your deepest connections fill you with love—one of the most potent positive emotions.

M = MEANING. Think of memories you hold dear. What makes your life full of meaning and purpose?

A = ACHIEVEMENT. Think about all the big and small "wins" of your life. What accomplishments make you proud, make you feel stronger, more confident?

When going through your bounce back, use PERMA as a gentle reminder that there are many different ways you can spiral up, enhance your well-being, and bounce back from bad things when they happen.

Bounce Back and Spiral Up

Happiness is all around you when you pause to notice its existence. Mindfulness raises your awareness of your surroundings and helps you become more connected to your thoughts and feelings. Even little things that typically go unnoticed because they are so routine, almost

Spiral Up

30 DAYS OF POSITIVE EMOTIONS

. . . .

Grab thirty note cards and a marker. On each note card write one simple, easy, doable idea for sparking positive energy. Include any activity you find enjoyable, but make sure you can easily accomplish any of your creative ideas on most days.

Positive Emotion Starters: Take a long walk, play catch with your dog, update your music playlists, rent a funny movie, go to the library, savor your morning coffee, call a friend, flip through photos, write a thank-you letter, buy fresh flowers, paint over an old canvas, send a greeting card, enjoy nature, get a pedicure, eat lunch outside, take a long bubble bath, or splurge on a treat you've been ogling.

Each day, draw a new card, do the activity, and take a moment to write about it in your journal. Repeat until you've been through all the cards. At the end of the month, see if you notice more positive emotions overall. What types of activities help you feel inspired, curious, kind, hopeful, connected, or proud? Note any particular activities that meant something to you. Consider including these more often and making them part of your bounce back plan.

fading into the background of your life, can become brighter, more colorful, more alive when you pause to notice the glimmers of happiness.

Search for small moments of happiness in the rituals of day-to-day life. For example, the next time you are washing dishes, take time to look out your kitchen window and appreciate the flowers in your backyard or pay special attention to the keepsakes on your windowsill. Where did they come from? What do they mean to you? Remind yourself that in many parts of the world, clean, running water is a luxury. On your drive to work, take time to notice the beauty of the sunshine peeking from behind the trees or listen to an inspiring podcast instead of the local news. These efforts don't have to be forced out of you like "Am I happy yet, dammit?" Each time you make a conscious choice to be present and appreciate something in the moment, it gives your spirit a gentle lift and adds to your happiness quotient for the day.

Three Good Things is an activity backed by research that shows you are more likely to experience positive emotions if you reflect daily on three good things in your life. Spend time with positive and inspiring people or create a "gratitude circle" of daily texts or emails with a private group of friends. Get in the habit of starting every journal entry with something you are grateful for, or keep a jar of "thankful thoughts" on your kitchen counter and encourage everyone in the family to add to it. Once the jar is full, read the contents together. Happiness grows from simple acts like greeting a stranger with a smile or paying for the next person's bus fare. These simple connections grow positive emotions and create an upward spiral of kindness that strengthens you emotionally.

Just like any other health habit, building positive emotions requires attention and effort. Prioritize and schedule a variety of activities you *think* will spark positive emotions on a regular basis. And don't be discouraged if your upward spirals don't always turn out how you expect them to. We're not in search of instant gratification here. The goal is to tip the scales toward positive emotions by spending increased amounts of time doing things we enjoy. More than just highlighting life's pleasurable moments, these upward spirals of energy can transform us for the better, opening our hearts and minds and creating a solid foundation for growing other body kindness habits. I hope your takeaways from this part of the book help you to have gratitude for all that your emotions do for you, and to remember that even when times are tough, it won't last forever.

BODY KINDNESS REFLECTION: Nobody is immune to bad things, but we all have the vaccination—resilience. At the start of this chapter I asked you to think about two bad things, one big and one small. Reread what you wrote. How are you already resilient? How would you like to bounce back in the future? How does practicing body kindness help you recover when bad things happen? Write your personal bounce back plan using what you've learned so far.

"I am not what happened to me. I am what I choose to become."

—Carl Gustav Jung

Part Three

Who You Are

Become Who You Want to Be

Chapter 8

Decide What You Stand for

Set Values-Driven Goals for Success

Philosophy

With every choice you make, you have the power to move closer to the life you want to live. When you set goals that are consistent with your personal values, you create an emotional connection with who you really are inside—the kind of person you want the world to see. You define what matters most to you and you put the plans in motion for success. Values-based living empowers positive decision-making and strengthens your ability to navigate obstacles. It works like this: Identify your values. Create meaningful goals. Use these values and goals to decide what committed actions you will take first. Finally, do what is needed to follow through on your commitments. This process is highly effective because it fosters creativity, engagement, and achievement—three powerful elements that contribute to a healthy well-being and a meaningful life.

BODY KINDNESS PILLARS
Living Your Values
Through Body Kindness

LOVE: Have the courage to set goals that reflect your values as an act of love.

CONNECT: Seek feedback from your body and mind that tells you whether or not you are living in line with your values.

CARE: Taking meaningful actions will transform you from the inside out.

Become Who You Want to Be

At this point you may be thinking, "I'm not sure how to make body kindness work in real life." If so, you're not alone. Many of my clients feel a little lost, stuck, or uncertain in the early days of their transformation. This chapter will provide the structure and guidance to help put your body kindness plans in motion. You will create new habits by intentionally setting goals based on what you want to stand for and how you want to behave. This approach may be very different from what you have tried in the past. **Body kindness goals are specific, realistic, and enjoyable *for you*!** You are committed to repeat actions over and over because you care about the outcome of accomplishing your goals.

Take a moment to get clear on the deeper meaning behind how you got to this point. Body kindness helps you create a better life for yourself. What that life looks like is up to you. Know this: Something very important to you is at stake. There are people and things you care about, deep in your heart. **This is bigger than looking a certain way.** There are meaningful changes you want to make because they matter to you—*Why?* What life are you missing out on because you've been stuck somewhere? What have you not been able to do? What regrets do you have? How badly do you want to change the voice in your head? Your *why* is full of emotion. It can be an uncomfortable reminder of what you

Spiral Up

I magine you are receiving a "lifetime achievement award." You're in a room filled with the people you love and respect. They are here to celebrate you and the unique gifts you bring to the world. Someone who is very close to you is on stage, presenting you with the award. Imagine what you would want them to say about your character—the kind of person you are, what you have meant to them. What might they say about your well-being? Write down these thoughts in your journal.

don't have, making you feel inadequate and unleashing thought bullies, and you try to hustle your way out of it. Answering the *why* gently is the body kindness thing to do. It supports love, connection, and caring for yourself. It helps uncover the meaning and purpose behind what you decide to do and how you'll do it.

People change. It's OK to say good-bye to the person you no longer want to be. You're still you at the core, but when you no longer want to identify with certain habits, when beliefs and behaviors are no longer serving to create a better life, it's your time to change. Make no mistake; this is your journey—your imperfect, unknown adventure. My hope is that now you will become your most open and creative self by using your personal values to guide you on this path. When your whole mindset shifts toward living a more authentic life, you become who you are meant to be. The revolution is already in progress. You don't have to wait for big things to happen. They already are!

Living Values Creates Change

Y our values constitute a way of being that matters to you. Once you reflect on your values and identify what is most important to you, you can set workable goals—things you have control over—to ensure that your self-care choices reinforce these values. You determine the actions you want to take to help you achieve your goals, and as you align goals with values, your new habits take shape. Your belief system is rock solid. When you can *clearly* see that choices you're making don't line up with your values, you think, "This isn't right!" and your motivation to make different decisions skyrockets. You want to take actions based on values. You just may have not realized when your choices are at odds with your values—until now!

Recall PACT, the acronym from Part Two (see page 114) that helps you take effective action. With PACT (Presence, Acceptance, Choice, Take action), you learned how to make the choices that matter most to you, even in the face of unhelpful thoughts and bad feelings. You learned that if you're conflicted about more than one choice option, that's OK. You can see two opposing choices and do what matters more. The more meaningful choice is aligned with your values—values that you are going to get back in touch with right now. Do you see the beauty, kindness, and love in this approach to creating a better life?

This structure is based on a type of therapy called Acceptance and Commitment Therapy (ACT), a mindfulness-based approach popularized by author and psychologist Dr. Russ Harris.

His books *The Happiness Trap* and *ACT Made Simple* were instrumental in helping me better understand how to help people change by working with their minds. Through ACT principles, my clients have overcome self-care obstacles such as sedentary lifestyles, poor body image, chronic dieting, and eating disorders. I have used ACT personally to tackle my most challenging body image issues, perfectionism, and emotional eating. In this therapy, you *accept* things you can't personally control while *committing* to take actions that will improve your quality of life. This means letting go of goals such as "fit into my old clothes" or "lose ten pounds before summer" and replacing them with a commitment to workable body kindness goals. Weight and inches aren't workable because you can't control them and create a better life for yourself. What matters are the steps you can take, like cooking at home, eating mindfully, and getting the sleep you need. These are actions you can track. All your efforts are mini-successes, giving you rewarding and satisfying pleasure along the way.

A Values Map to Your New Habits

Asking "What kind of person do I want to become?" and "What is most important to me?" is the fastest way to resolve any inner barriers that stand between you and the life you want to live.

Grab your journal or a notebook and complete these activities by hand.

You may want to do these by yourself entirely, or do them with someone you care about. Studies suggest that talking about your values helps strengthen your connection to them. Working with a buddy can also help you push through discomfort, self-doubt, or (gasp) wanting to skip these steps! You and a friend or small group of friends may find this energizing, therapeutic, and more informative than if you tried on your own.

Step One: Identify Your Values

Pick one area of well-being you would like to start with. From here you will create one value, one goal, and a short list of actions. Below are suggestions to help you get started:

- Food
- Fitness/exercise
- Sleep
- Fun/leisure
- Thoughts and feelings
- Relationships/socializing
- Mindfulness
- Caring and nurturing (self and others)

Now come up with one value that connects you to this area of your life. You can brainstorm several options and then choose one if you would like. You can always come back to more values later.

Complete this statement: *I want to be a person who _____ [insert value].*

Here are just a few possible values to get your mind brimming with ideas.

- I want to be a person who *eats mindfully.*
- I want to be a person who *cooks regularly.*
- I want to be a person who *exercises consistently.*
- I want to be a person who *gets enough sleep.*
- I want to be a person who *volunteers.*
- I want to be a person who *makes time for fun.*
- I want to be a person who *speaks kindly to herself.*
- I want to be a person who *invests in valued relationships.*

Keep in mind that a value is a "way of being" that you can control. Behaviors, choices, and actions in pursuit of a better life align with values. Feelings cannot be values because you can't control them. If you come up with "feeling" words, look at the story behind each feeling. For example, consider the value "I want to be a person who *feels comfortable having my picture taken.*" Reframe your value by writing what you would be striving toward if you were working on feeling comfortable: "I want to be a person who *accepts herself as she is in the present moment.*" In this example, you may still feel uncomfortable having your picture taken, but you're willing to be in the photo by practicing self-acceptance. And just in case you're wondering, weighing a certain amount or fitting into old clothes aren't values.

....

Step Two: Discover the Meaning of Your Value

....

Choose one value statement and write about it. Finding meaning boosts your motivation, helps you identify problems, and reveals options for goals.

- Why is this value important to you?

- How do you nurture this value in your life now?

- What is challenging about living this value now?

- How will you remember your values when you need to?

Here's an example. The value is "nourishing my body."

I want to be a person who nourishes my body because I want to be healthy. I want to live a long time and I want to enjoy my life. I need energy to get through the day so I can do my job and take care of the people I love (these values are most important to me). I know that when I take time to plan and eat balanced meals, I have more energy and I feel better. One of my biggest challenges to nourishing my body is making the time to sit and enjoy a meal. If I'm by myself, I'm more likely to

just grab something and eat on the run. However, if I put a little time into planning, I have foods on hand that make it easier for me to eat well every day. I'm more likely to eat well if I have a healthy lunch ready to just dig in to. When I want to put off goals that support nourishing my body, I will remember my value by thinking about my houseplants. When I neglect my plants they look sad, shriveled, and weak. I'll imagine myself as one of my plants not getting what it needs to grow and thrive. I'll say to myself—it's time to nourish yourself.

Values don't come easy to everyone. If you'd like to explore them in a different way, you can try two other approaches: *interview yourself* and *write your story.*

INTERVIEW YOURSELF TO IDENTIFY YOUR VALUES

....

Pretend you are interviewing yourself. You can even use the "empty chair" form of therapy. (It's a real thing! Google "empty chair technique.") Sit in one chair as an interviewer to ask the question. Switch to the other chair to answer it. Here are some questions to get you started:

- What matters to you most?

- How do you hope your life will be different in a few years from now?

- What are rules you live by?

- How would your friends describe what you live for?

WRITE YOUR STORY TO IDENTIFY YOUR VALUES

Values offer the opportunity for you to tell your future story. Writing, storytelling, and journaling are very effective at generating ideas, building courage, and answering questions as you muddle through uncertainty. Here are just a few ways you can try writing your story that may give you clues to your values in other meaningful ways.

Write a thank-you letter from your future self. What is she telling you about what life is like now that you have changed, and what you did to get there?

Dear Kate,

All I can say is you amaze me. You have come a long way the past year. You used to obsess over your weight, track your calories in a spreadsheet, compare yourself to everyone else, and you were absolutely miserable. No matter how hard you worked, it wasn't good enough. But through your commitment to finding real health, you have healed your relationship with your body and food. You don't judge yourself based on the scale anymore. You trust yourself to eat balanced meals without calorie counting, thanks to following your hunger. You finally said, "It's OK to eat dessert!" and now you do so with your husband. You are so much happier and confident, Kate. You have always been beautiful, but now you are starting to believe how amazing you are, inside and out.

Write your "mission statement" about your life, describing your purpose, hopes, and dreams.

Read your "lifetime achievement award" brainstorm from the opening of this chapter and craft your acceptance speech.

Any one of these approaches is bound to elicit useful information for you to get inspired by your values and lead to effective goal setting.

Walking Backward— What's Really in Your Way?

You might have noticed that by doing the writing exercises you identify problems in your life that you would like to fix and hidden obstacles that are getting in your way. You may even have quite a list in your journal from previous activities in this book. This is useful information for the next steps of setting values-based goals and taking effective actions. Now is a great time for you to revisit this work and the body kindness manifesto for inspiration.

When I want to explore the source of a problem, I call it *walking backward*. It's a way of tracking back to the start of your concerns in order to put workable goals and actions in place. Ask the question, "What happened that led to this problem?" As you learn more, you start to uncover a more complete understanding of what's happening in your life. This is just mindfulness, nothing more. You shouldn't try to figure out everything, just take some time to see your life's picture a little more clearly.

Along with your values assessment, this information can guide you toward a more meaningful life, serving as a moral compass for the choices you make and the boundaries you may need to set in order to succeed. Anna came to my office fully aware that she was eating and drinking too much in an attempt to manage her anxiety. Her concerns were exacerbated by the broken promises she had made to herself to make up for her mistakes—go for a punishing run, eat just an apple at lunch—which ultimately led to her self-sabotaging actions. We looked at what she was doing that was in conflict with her values and identified ways to realign. Through this process, we uncovered that she had a lot of difficulty setting boundaries. This prompted Anna to commit to one action: "Speak up when something is bothering me." This simple resolution required her to stay diligent regarding boundaries on a daily basis. "I am very much a work in progress on this front. I don't always get the thoughts out of my mouth, but in my head, I am much quicker to identify why a situation is leading to anxiety and the proper way to resolve it. This simple change has helped me stay away from other 'comfort' solutions like alcohol and food."

Creating Goals That Work

With a value statement and narrative in hand, you can begin to think about workable goals—things you can control that are in line with your values and help you create a better life. You can think of goals and actions as going together. As you pick goals, you'll identify actions that help you achieve them. There are any number of actions you can come up with based on what you've already learned in this book. All you have to do is choose.

It's not about being right or wrong. All actions that serve your goals are good actions.

I don't want to downplay the significance of committed actions. Power is a potent ingredient. It comes from within your own mind and body. When you take committed actions, you are powerful. You can conquer your own thoughts and feelings; you can overcome all the odds you're fighting. You are stronger than you think. Know this going into it, because right now, as you think about goals and actions, you're probably hearing one of those voices in your head criticizing, judging, "should"-ing all over you. Just notice them, say "hello," and go on your merry way, exuding your awesome prowess in goal setting. You are a warrior. Raise up those arms, beat on your chest, and stay focused on this important work. Unhelpful voices cannot get in your way unless you let them.

I have three guidelines to help you create workable goals: 1) Choose only goals you that interest you. 2) Set goals that are challenging. 3) Don't set a dead person's goal.

Choose Only Goals That Interest You

The worst kind of goal you can set is the one you "should" do because someone suggested it to you or you feel you have to do because everyone else seems to be doing it. Don't bother with anything that does not appeal to you. Life is too short and there are too many other options to be bored. Do what you care about. You'll have much more fun and you'll feel those upward spirals. There is so much power in the phrase "Nope. Not for me." The goals you will accomplish are the ones you find most interesting. If you hear yourself saying, "This is hard, but totally fun" or "I can't wait until the next time I get to do that," then you know you're on the right track.

Set Goals That Are Challenging

Create goals with various levels of difficulty. This is important to provide a unique combination of finding early success, staying engaged, and opening yourself up to awe-inspiring possibilities that can change you. All three of these types of goals help you in their own way. Some people find thinking creatively about goals motivating. Others find it overwhelming. Do what works for you. All you need to take a chance is one goal with one supporting action. When you start with one small change, it gets easier to build and grow from there, moving to the next level of challenge.

I put challenging goals into three categories—desires, dreams, and dares. *Desire goals* are fun "no-brainers"—goals you know you'll enjoy and accomplish.

You'll get a boost of motivation with early successes on desire goals. Now add some goals that will make you work a little bit. Goals that require more effort often carry bigger rewards. I call these *dream goals*. Then there are *dare goals*. These goals feel one step beyond your reach. You have the most uncertainty about achieving dare goals, but just thinking about them feels exhilarating. These special goals stretch you to imagine your best possible self.

Dare goals tend to be life-changing, meaningful experiences. Of course they require the most effort, but even if you never fully achieve them, they can still keep you in touch with the sense of wonder and purpose that helped create them. And by keeping your wildest dreams close to your heart, you open the door for unexpected smaller desires and dreams along the way. Each time you accomplish a desire or dream goal, it puts you one step (and one thought) closer to your big dare goals!

Don't Set a Dead Person's Goal

Dead people will "never eat sugar again," "never eat bagels at office parties," and "never order Chinese food at 10 p.m." Restraining goals like these actually communicate to your brain to do the very thing you wish to avoid. Scientists have studied this phenomenon, called "ironic rebound effect," and found dieters to be the most vulnerable. They discovered that the more you try to suppress a desire, the more frequently and intensely thoughts arise. Thoughts can quickly get overwhelming and tire out the part of your brain that manages your self-control. As your mind hammers at you, "Don't eat the chocolate. Don't eat the chocolate! DON'T EAT THE CHOCOLATE!" you try even harder to suppress the thoughts, and the urge to succumb to them intensifies. If your mental resources to fight this urge are maxed out, such as when you're tired, it's late in the day, or you've been thinking about avoiding it too long, you're more likely to give in. It's like an arm wrestling match between the Incredible Hulk and Pee-wee Herman.

You can outsmart the ironic rebound effect by setting a goal that reflects a positive action you can take. Instead of vowing to never eat sweets, flip the focus and ask yourself, "How would I like to act?" Think about what you would do in place of the habit you're trying to avoid. Your desire to stop eating candy from the break room becomes "I'd like to keep working and consider eating sweets later, when I can actually enjoy them. For now, I'll savor the sweetness of my coffee and stay focused on my deadlines."

Choose Your Desires, Dreams, and Dares

Now that you have criteria for your goals and actions, write them down. The following example includes a desire, a dream, and a dare goal from an actual client session. The client's initial value was "I want to be a person who feels confident with her food choices." Since she used off-limits "feeling" words (you can't control feelings) she reframed her value to a workable action. She decided that if she felt more confident with her food choices, one of the things she would be striving to do is make committed efforts to choose healthy foods. Her present behavior consisted of inadequate meal planning and many "screw it" spontaneous food choices more representative of her fatigue and frustration with her behavior than her real food preferences and desires to nourish herself better.

VALUE: I want to become a person who *nourishes her body.*

GOAL: Prepare a balanced plate (a *desire*).

ACTIONS: Make weekly grocery lists with a variety of fruits and vegetables. Prep snacks ahead of time when unpacking groceries.

GOAL: Take a healthful cooking class (a *dream*).

ACTIONS: Look up classes this week. Watch online videos this weekend for self-teaching.

GOAL: Travel to another country as a "foodie" (a *dare*).

ACTIONS: This month, read books and talk to people who have done it. Test out a new recipe or visit a restaurant from a region I'd like to visit someday.

Danielle had a list of goals a mile long. She wanted to quit drinking, smoking, and emotional eating all at the same time—but instead of trying to limit these behaviors, we decided to identify what values were important to her and create goals that would reflect that. Friends are really important to Danielle, so one of the first things we identified as a value was her desire to spend more time with positive influences. Then she also shared that it was important to her to eat more healthfully and exercise regularly. In the past Danielle embraced the identity of the "happy fat girl." She was the life of every party and used her sense of humor to connect with people. When we first started working together, she had no idea how to be a different person and was afraid she would lose friends in the process. **But while she desperately wanted support from friends, she wanted to live an authentic life even more.** Eventually she felt strong enough to say, "If people leave me, I'll just have to live with it. I don't want to be the girl who cares more about being *fun enough* than taking good care of herself." Once we shifted her focus toward the values of true friendship, healthy food choices, and more movement, Danielle learned that she could still have fun with many of her friends and work toward her goals. And she also made new friends and strengthened some relationships in the process. She learned that she was interesting in more ways than she realized and began creating habits that satisfied her—like hiking, completing a 5K, and trying out new recipes on her friends and family.

Your personal values are an infinitely powerful catalyst for change. Once your values and decisions are aligned, a quick gut-check is the fastest way to stay on track toward whatever goals you hope to achieve. You can quickly refocus your energy and choices whenever necessary because your inner compass is a reliable guide. Values can motivate and inspire you. Honoring them will keep you spiraling up in mood and energy and will light the way when the right path is unclear. Your values can be a source of strength and affirmation when you're having difficulty. This also gives you a unique, measurable way to celebrate successes along the way. Because, in the end, success is not about whether you actually reach any goal you set out to achieve, but whether you're living a life you feel proud of.

BODY KINDNESS REFLECTION: Open up your journal and spend fifteen minutes thinking about your values and goals. In what ways are you not living the values you identified as important to you? On a scale of 1 to 10, how ready are you to change these habits? How confident are you? How will you *remember your values* when you need them to focus your committed actions?

> "Find out who you are and do it on purpose."
>
> —Dolly Parton

Chapter 9

Transform Your Health with Action

Planning and Time Management for Success

Philosophy

If the secret to transforming your health lies in taking committed actions, then understanding how to stay focused and driven toward your goals is essential. You don't have unlimited time, money, energy, or brainpower. These resources can easily get wasted without a plan that suits you. The body kindness plan helps you stay mindful and motivated, with visual reminders and simplified ways to organize yourself.

BODY KINDNESS PILLARS
Living Your Values with Body Kindness

LOVE: Show yourself love by respecting your most precious resources—time, money, and energy.

CONNECT: When you take action, your mind and body will signal what's working and tell you if your plan needs attention.

CARE: Through upward spirals, your new committed actions begin to take hold, and caring for yourself gets easier and more enjoyable.

The Body Kindness Blueprint

With values, goals, and actions in hand, you have almost everything you need to drive upward spirals and transform your health from the inside out. Instead of seeing all these things you want to do as individual parts, look at them as part of an integrated *self-care system* of things that are important to you. This might include food, fitness, sleep, socializing, and making special time with loved ones. Even if you don't tackle everything (and I recommend you don't), by observing how all of your goals are wired together you'll see a more complete picture of your challenges, generate ideas for your action plan, and figure out the choices that suit you best to form lasting habits. I do this with every new client by creating a *body kindness blueprint*. Starting with a blank piece of paper, I draw a circle with their name on it at the center. As they share their personal story, I take notes and draw more circles to create a visual guide we can use for planning.

When my client Sheryl came to her first session, she was extremely frustrated with herself and expressed significant doubt that she could succeed at changing. Her primary health concerns were recent weight gain and lab results that showed high blood sugar and cholesterol. She frequently stayed late at work, only to arrive home to an empty house, now that her kids were grown and she was divorced. Exhausted and lonely, she didn't want to put effort into dinner and instead reached for chips, ice cream, and other snacks she "saved" for emotional eating. She was full of remorse and

Spiral Up

I magine the time fairy granted you an extra day to your week—a magical eighth day nobody else has. What would you do with that time? Write down as many ideas as you can come up with, no matter how far-fetched they may seem. Put a star next to ideas that energize you the most.

fearing things could get worse, she desperately wanted to take action on all the things she knew she should be doing. As I put together her body kindness blueprint, we talked about boundaries. She admitted that she's a perfectionist, rarely feels like her efforts are adequate, and finds it difficult to say no to various requests. She's always staying late at work because there's so much to do. Instead of socializing at the gym or asking a friend to go for a walk after work, she stays tethered to her office chair. While Sheryl enjoys many different healthful foods, she has been a dieter her whole life. She finds her short list of "allowed" foods boring. She enjoyed cooking for her family, but when I ask about preparing dinner for herself, she says "Hmph, I don't want to." She usually grocery shops on a whim and typically buys prepackaged foods and snacks she has difficulty eating in moderation. She even compared it to feeling like an alcoholic who couldn't stop buying beer. "Why do I put this food in the cart knowing I'm going to reach for it when I don't feel like taking care of myself?" She wondered.

I asked Sheryl how she handles her feelings aside from eating, and she responded, "I don't have feelings. Well, I know I have feelings, but I don't have time to feel them." What would happen if Sheryl took a moment to acknowledge feeling tired, frustrated, and overworked? Instead of emotional eating, she could do something nice for herself like cook something interesting or enjoy a good meal out.

Sheryl's body kindness blueprint revealed that she wasn't managing her time to include eating well and exercising. As we accounted for every hour of her day, she clearly saw that she needed to leave work at a more reasonable time. Enjoying pleasant evenings would help boost her mood and energy, decreasing the chance of being triggered to eat emotionally. Using the balanced plate as a guide, we brainstormed ideas for delicious and easy dinners. Although she was not enthusiastic about cooking again, she knew she could be eventually. Sheryl decided to leave chips and ice cream off the grocery list. "I just need a break. I want to get

SHERYL'S BLUEPRINT
BODY KINDNESS AT WORK

Sheryl's blueprint identifies her unique plans to change.

Sheryl

SELF-COMPASSION
Journal daily, read body kindness manifesto when I need a boost.

HOBBIES
Once a month, make progress on a fun goal—a painting class, making your own cheese, knitting a scarf, etc.

SLEEP
Get ready for bed by 9 p.m. Read in bed until 9:30 to get 8 hours of sleep.

SOCIAL
One dinner per week with a friend, exercise classes, one weekend social activity.

TIME
Leave work on time. Stick to the schedule, no matter what!

FOOD
Meal plan properly, shop from a list, use "three-legged stool" thinking, include foods I love.

FITNESS
Three exercise classes per week, walk 10,000 steps a day on weekends, focus on health benefits, not weight loss.

in the habit of overcoming that urge to eat those foods when I'm feeling tired and lonely."

When we reviewed her body kindness blueprint, Sheryl could clearly see her self-care system at work. The combination of poor sleep, working too long, and isolating herself suppressed her energy and mood, making it difficult to establish good self-care routines. The plan we developed consisted of actions that would help keep her spiraling up with positive emotions, such as the endorphins from a workout, energy from better sleep, and satisfaction from being social. She recognized that "Ms. Perfectionist" was exhausting her brain, making her feel bad, and sabotaging her motivation. She needed to cultivate a more compassionate inner voice to stick up for herself and take back her evenings—a voice that says, "It's time to turn off the computer and get dressed for your workout."

After only a few weeks of constructing body kindness blueprints, Sheryl told me the progress was remarkable. "When I leave work on time, I exercise. The energy I feel makes me actually want to cook something good. I know we aren't supposed to focus on weight loss, but my clothes are getting looser. I'm not dieting. I'm eating *more*, and I'm taking care of my whole self. I'm still tempted to emotionally eat, but the tools are working." Three months later her labs showed improved cholesterol and blood sugar. All in all, she lost about ten pounds, which she said was close to what she gained when her emotional eating spiraled out of control. Now she's working on accepting her body. "I won't go back, but I'm having a hard time letting this be my body. I have decades of dieting and body shaming to unravel and I'm not there yet. I'm a work in progress!"

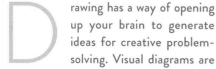

Create Your Body Kindness Blueprint

Drawing has a way of opening up your brain to generate ideas for creative problem-solving. Visual diagrams are helpful for you to see a bigger picture and anticipate obstacles to your routines. They also serve as a useful tool for planning your time and the actions you want to take. Don't worry—you're not scheduling anything—yet! You're taking a focused look at how you spend your time and then you're drawing a picture of it.

. . . .

1 Describe your typical day in words. Account for every hour, from the time you wake up through the time you fall asleep, noting how many hours you usually get—is it enough? Describe what you're doing, and how you generally feel throughout the day, particularly noting the times you catch yourself feeling hungry, bored, tired, or bad. Read over your entire day, noting your concerns. Do you stop and eat when you feel hungry? When do you drink water, coffee, or alcohol? Think about events most likely to lead to downward spirals, not every little fear you have about change. Ask yourself: Why is this challenging? What else is happening that concerns me? Can you spot triggers that seem to cause you to skip workouts, eat emotionally, or stay up too late? What is likely to prevent you from taking action on the goals that matter to you? Write as much detail as you need to really understand your obstacles. For example, when thinking about exercise, you might note feeling tired and lack of time. For food, you might dislike cooking or cleaning up the mess and you really don't like vegetables very much.

You may want to repeat this activity for a typical weekend. You're done with this activity when you have a sense for how you're spending your time and how you might navigate obstacles to take successful action toward your goals.

. . . .

2 Draw your body kindness blueprint. With your values and goals from the last chapter and a good sense of how you spend your time, draw your blueprint. I recommend you start with food, fitness, sleep, and fun. Draw your name in a circle and then draw connecting circles with ideas for committed actions below. It's important that you notice the relationship of your behavior patterns. How is taking an action on a sleep goal going to help you with the others? Hopefully, you're feeling more motivated and confident as you put together your plan. But you might also feel uncertainty, like "yeah right, how am I going to get all this done in my schedule?" Instead of becoming overwhelmed, imagine the best possible action you can take right now to deal with your challenges and write that down. It should fit your view of body kindness: interesting or enjoyable, helps you spiral up in energy and feel better, and is achievable now.

Your body kindness blueprint is a visual reminder of your values and goals. It can help you schedule activities and make it easier to track your progress with all your actions listed in one place. Keep the blueprint simple and manageable. If it's not useful, then it's too complicated. Your drawing should feel "just right." You're taking on enough to challenge yourself.

Avoid the overwhelming feeling of "too much" by scaling back. You can make a new blueprint each week, or as you need to create new visual reminders of what is important to you. Taking *any* positive action in line with your values (no matter how small) is the correct next step.

Planning Your Accomplishments

You're going to be successful in transforming your health just like any other "big" accomplishment in life—by planning it and staying committed to the plan. Give yourself a reasonable amount of time each week to plan *when* you will take action, line up *what* you need, and *write* it all down in a schedule you intend to follow. This will remind you of your commitments and keep you mindful of your progress. It also allows you a chance to change your mind, try something different, or refine your plan to best suit you week to week.

I have a saying for committed actions: "Do it for day two." Bring all your commitment to day two. Day one gets all the glory of your focused attention and day two is easily forgotten about. This is a problem for learning habits because you need the repetition. Think about how you feel after accomplishing a workout goal. You show up day one, full of self-doubt. You finish it. Chances are it wasn't as bad as you thought it would be, you felt better afterward, and you're proud of your accomplishment. But be mindful if the self-congratulations is cueing you to take a break: "I did it yesterday so I'll skip today." It might seem like a reasonable and rational choice. It also could be rewarding—a chance to avoid discomfort or just do something else with your time. Imagine if your goal was day two and doing the exercise again was the challenge and the reward. Go ahead and tweak your activity, the duration or intensity of exercise; just don't skip it altogether. Practice your commitment to your goals as often as your schedule allows. Practice observing your thoughts talking you out of taking action, and do it anyway. Future days get easier as your habit takes hold. In fact, you'll start to "crave" exercise, sleep, and balanced plates. But you need to give your brain a chance to learn through repetition.

An effective plan needs to work for you. Be honest about your personality (e.g., late sleeper or late worker) and take that into account as you make decisions on how you'll spend your resources, the big ones being time, money, and energy. Consider your environment. How can you *spiral up* your space to make life easier, reduce distractions, and slash your thinking time? How will you avoid choice traps so you make the decisions you really want? Later in this chapter, I share organization tips to help save time and money on your daily food and fitness plans.

Once you see how all of your body kindness goals impact one another, you will recognize the value of committing to daily actions that support them. Sheryl was known to rebel, even against herself. In order to keep her focused on her plan, I asked her to write a letter to herself about her goals and why they were important to her. She explained what she wanted to achieve and how *not* meeting those goals impacts her well-being negatively. She told herself she would succeed and described her future self after achieving her goals. She took the letter out before going grocery shopping or after a tough workday to help her remember her values and stay committed to her goals.

Over the years Sheryl had tried Weight Watchers, Jenny Craig, Nutrisystem, and more—anything she thought might help take the weight off. Working together with the body kindness blueprint, we developed an understanding of *why* she was doing what she was doing. She couldn't just count calories or avoid certain foods, she needed to assess who she truly wanted to be and commit to working toward becoming that person. She needed to start acting in line with her goals and her dreams. Sheryl's plan became the compass for her new destination, away from diets and toward the practice of body kindness. Your plan is only successful if it helps you take action. If you don't write it down, it's not likely to happen. Inevitably, you need to take a good look at your schedule and figure out how you will accomplish your goals.

The Myth of Busyness
(You Have More Time Than You Think)

Creating the life you want requires both intention and attention. While the steps you take can undoubtedly be squeezed into smaller and shorter units of time, figuring out the best use of your time requires effort. Sometimes the fear of not being able to succeed can mask itself with statements like "I can't handle this! I don't have the time!" If you have ever felt like your time is not your own, or if you think a lack of time is keeping you from living the life you want, restructure your time to make room for what's most important to you.

In her bestselling book *Overwhelmed: Work, Love, and Play When No One Has the Time*, author Brigid Schulte explores why Americans are so committed to being "busy," and how their lives suffer as a result. She deconstructs a surprising reality that researchers have discovered: Busyness has become a bragging right, a status symbol we flaunt to friends, coworkers, and family indicating our value and worth in society. She says we have come to loathe idleness and view leisure as unnecessary and wasteful. However, researchers argue we actually don't understand the benefits leisure provides. We trivialize leisure, and this interferes with our health and happiness as a culture. Simply defined, leisure is free time to do something you enjoy. Technically, almost everything you do for body kindness could be seen as leisure, if you choose activities that you enjoy. It's time to start seeing *that* as an accomplishment. Schulte was shocked when a time use researcher said she, like most Americans, had about thirty hours a week of leisure time. She likened her days to time confetti—scattered bits and scraps of "to-do's" and no real satisfying sense of how she spent her time. She says part of the problem is driven by workplaces that aren't family friendly and competition among moms. We have to

do it all, have it all, and be it all (serious FOMO). Detach yourself from the idea that busyness is a badge of honor. You may be a busy person, but you don't have to be overwhelmed and your health shouldn't have to suffer. While we wait for our culture to change, let's not sit idly. Let's make good use of the time we have. Even if looks like confetti, let's throw ourselves one hell of a body kindness party!

Give Your Schedule a Body Kindness Makeover

My method for **time management** is straightforward. You are going to release yourself from any unhelpful narratives regarding what it means to be a good mother, spouse, colleague, friend, etc. and take back one of the most powerful resources you possess—your time. You will do this by setting boundaries for your time, based on what is essential and what is most important to you. Here are five steps to help you get started:

1 Clear the clutter.

2 Make a list of "keeping the household together" tasks.

3 Schedule what you *must* do.

4 Schedule what you *want* to do.

5 Learn the beautiful, complete sentence of "No."

CLEAR THE CLUTTER

It's time to take out the trash! With your body kindness blueprint and calendar handy, start de-cluttering. Make a "to-don't list." Think about the lingering things that are just distracting you and overwhelming you. They don't serve a value or a goal, and really, the only reason they are hanging on is because of some kind of guilt. Let it go. Scratch it. Delete it. What are your time wasters? Too much TV, social media, or even cleaning and organizing—is your world really going to crumble if your closet doesn't look like Marie Kondo's? We all have projects that are important, but if you've been putting off self-care for a year because you're too busy restoring your furniture, then you have a problem with your priorities. Get rid of time wasters. Everything that remains on your list is a potential distraction, drain on mental energy, and time suck. You're already dealing with a time shortage and you can't afford to be wasteful. Do not skip this step. You need to make space if you want to take action. You will continue to clear clutter off your plate as you move forward with the next steps.

KEEPING THE HOUSEHOLD TOGETHER

Whether you're a household of one, two, or many, it's high time everyone under the same roof worked together to get things done. Start from the time the first person wakes up until the last person goes to bed and create a list of *essential* household tasks for your busiest times of day, usually the morning, evening, and weekends. For example: wake up, make coffee and breakfast, feed and take out the dogs, wake kids, get ready for work, pack lunches, check backpacks, get out the door. Your evening routine may look similar and include everything from dinner to clean up and help with homework. You will eventually divide the effort or create a manageable schedule if you're on your own. Make sure your final to-do list has only essentials—eating, sleeping, some cleaning, and getting people where they need to be. If something is important but not a daily essential, like laundry, groceries, or bills, put it on the weekend list.

SCHEDULE WHAT YOU *MUST* DO

With some wiggle room in your calendar, start to fill up space with your body kindness actions and other things in life that only you can do. Only you can do your exercise, only you can get your teeth cleaned. Maybe you have to be at work during designated hours or you have to pick up your kids from school at a specific time. Put all of these things on your calendar to get a real sense of what your day of "musts" looks like.

Now is the time to get specific. You might decide you need to set a reminder on your work calendar so you leave on time. Maybe you go to bed earlier to wake up for an early morning workout or start work earlier so you can leave with enough evening time to do what's important. Maybe you schedule your lunch break—and take it. This is when you'll slap on some sneakers and enjoy a walk outside followed by a brief lunch before going back to work. When you incorporate body kindness actions into your calendar as non-negotiable events, then you won't catch yourself trying to squeeze them in at inopportune times or skipping them altogether. This also helps people in your life know when you're available and when you're not. And by blocking out your schedule this way, you may discover pockets of time you didn't see before. Before moving on make sure at least some, if not all, of your body kindness blueprint is accounted for in your "musts."

SCHEDULE WHAT YOU WANT TO DO—AND DELEGATE THE REST!

Now go back to the "keeping the household together" list and take first dibs at things you actually enjoy—or prefer

not to delegate—and get them in your personal calendar. Maybe you decide you want to lead the meal planning, grocery shopping, and most of the cooking. Delegate the cleaning, laundry, trash, and odds-and-ends errands. Put more time than you think these activities will take because they always take longer than you anticipate. I usually schedule three hours over a weekend to meal plan, shop, and prep ahead. I swear by my family "business" meetings. Once a week my husband and I sit down to our bacon and waffle breakfast while the girls watch cartoons and we run through our list to shore up the next week's schedule. We get to clear both our heads of worry as we divvy up household responsibilities, make sure we each get our "me time," and let lower priority "nice to haves" fall off the list until next week. Even if you do these meetings once a month, you can keep your worries in a Word document rather than floating in your head, where they will likely turn into thought bullies. If delegating is hard for you, look at it another way. This is part of your job as a parent and partner—setting boundaries and working together. Kids need to learn personal responsibility and life skills. Even very young ones can help here and there. They know how to pick up toys. Just because you can do it faster doesn't mean you should do it. Keep in mind everyone needs time to adjust to the new schedule until it becomes normal. You worry about *you* first. Don't allow yourself to get distracted by other things that aren't on your list. When the inevitable hiccup happens, use that information to correct course at the next business meeting. Expect everyone will make mistakes and the household operations will be messy as you begin to take back your time and make room for body kindness.

LEARN THE BEAUTIFUL, COMPLETE SENTENCE OF "NO"

Many of us fail to realize that "No" is a complete sentence. When it comes to body kindness, harnessing the power of this word can be transformative. As you look over the "must do" and "want to do" calendar you've outlined for yourself, it becomes necessary to leave out any activities that don't match your body kindness goals and necessary responsibilities. One quick way to gauge if you really want to do something is to ask yourself the question, "What will I be saying no to if I say yes to this?" For example, one friend limited the number of activities she volunteered for at her kids' school when she realized that all the bake sales and room parties were cutting into the actual time she spent with her family. "Sorry, honey, Mommy can't read you a book right now. I have to finish this Excel spreadsheet for the Scholastic Book Fair/Box Tops for Education/Holiday Shop." Another way to keep the "Yes Monster" in check is by reminding yourself that "not now" doesn't mean "not ever." Consider taking a temporary break from distractions out of respect for your body kindness goals that are important to you. If you still have room in your calendar after all this scheduling, *hurray!* Make sure you didn't forget downtime or fun times with friends and family, or go back to your values and goals and schedule time for one of your *dream* or *dare* goals.

TAKE YOUR TIME FINDING TIME

Time schedules can take months to hit a groove. Be patient with this transformation. If you're still overwhelmed by time management and worried about what won't get done, commit to a two-week experiment with your new schedule. It might just be pessimism, and you need a chance to test-drive the new routine before making any other decisions. Or it could be a wake-up call that even after taking steps to clear the clutter and saying no, you still don't take action on your body kindness goals. Is "Ms. Perfectionist" calling the shots? I don't think it's realistic to expect our schedules to be effortless. You're still busy. The difference is you feel some freedom and space to take action. Are you falling into "choice traps?" Get curious about why you aren't following through on your goals. Is time still to blame? For some people, the key to saving time is outsourcing—this means paying someone else to do a task and create more time for everyone. Far too often I've seen clients with the financial means for a house-keeper or investing in meal delivery kits a few days a week, but they feel guilty about spending the money. Instead, they remain stressed and their goals are stagnant. Outsourcing is not an answer for everybody, but if the only reason you won't try it is because you *should* be able to do it all, reconsider those expectations. Regardless if outsourcing solves some of your time woes or not, we can all improve our time efficiency and save money practicing body kindness.

Save Time, Save Money, and Eat Well

Money concerns are a major source of stress, and a whopping 70 percent of people live paycheck to paycheck. Stretching our dollars is a necessity for most of us. When it comes to eating well, affordability is one of the consistent barriers for many people. It's a myth that eating healthy is expensive. You don't have to buy a $10 cold-pressed green juice to get vegetables! Eggs are 15 cents apiece and pulses are a powerful source of protein and fiber, ounce for ounce costing one-tenth the price of beef. By and large, making your own meals most of the time is better for you and doesn't have to cost a lot. My plan will help you slash food waste by making good use of what you already have. You'll fatten your pocketbook and bring together your food odds and ends, making balanced meals happen for a song. And I have tips to help you do it quickly.

TIME/MONEY SAVER #1: MEAL PLAN FOR THE WEEK

The key to saving money on food is setting a budget and buying only what you need from the store. In order to make that happen, you need to plan your menu, make a list, and stick to it. Meal planning once a week also helps you avoid the midweek chaos of "what's for dinner" that leads to dialing expensive food delivery or wasting time on a harried grocery store run.

Start with a commitment to making the balanced plate happen. That's your meal plan checklist—fruit, vegetable, whole grain, protein—check! I always start my meal plan by using what I already have. As you search through your refrigerator, freezer, and pantry, make two lists, your menu and grocery list. Here's a culinary secret: You really can't mess up balanced plates. You can make breakfast for dinner. Leftovers from Monday and Tuesday can be served together for dinner Wednesday. Even if you don't have lettuce, any combination of fresh vegetables chopped up counts as a salad. Add beans and salad dressing, pesto, or lemon and olive oil and some fruit on the side—that's a meal! Think of it as an experiment. If you're a recipe person and you need ideas, search online as you discover what you have on hand. The website Supercook.com lets you enter ingredients and shares recipes from the most popular cooking websites. As you complete your menu, make sure your grocery list has only the items you need to finish the meals to save time and money at the store.

LEFTOVERS, REIMAGINED

Leftovers last about four days in the refrigerator. Before you trash them, reinvent a new dish and save your money.

RICE from Chinese takeout—Microwave it and top with a fried egg and add any cooked vegetables you have on hand.

VEGETABLES—Reheat them in a skillet, add beaten eggs, and cook until set.

CHICKEN OR STEAK—Turn them into a casserole or strata. Toss the chunks of meat with veggies and cubed bread. Add beaten eggs and milk and bake at 350°F until set.

MEXICAN—Wrap your leftover fillings in a tortilla with a scrambled egg. Top with avocado, cheese, beans, and salsa verde or taco sauce.

ITALIAN—Turn your leftover sauce and meatballs into personal pizzas. Top pita with sauce, meat, vegetables, and cheese and bake for 10 minutes at 350°F.

If you can't use your leftovers within four days, freeze them. Write the date on the package and plan to use them within a month. Your freezer can become a money-saving machine. Surprising foods that freeze well include milk, shredded cheese, raw eggs, bread, fresh herbs blended in olive oil and garlic in ice cube trays, portions of unused sauces and canned foods, and most vegetables and fruits—to name a few. Wrap your food well using freezer paper, plastic wrap, foil, freezer storage bags, or plastic or glass containers, removing as much air as possible.

TIME/MONEY SAVER #2: SHOP FROM YOUR LIST

Keep calm and stick to your list—for the most part. For example, if you're planning to cook green beans, but the asparagus looks better or offers a surprising deal, go with the asparagus. Remember, if you buy too much you create more work for yourself. You'll have more food to organize and more food that could go bad on you. Be a shopping minimalist to maximize your time and money savings. I love a good deal, but don't get too carried away with sales, especially if your cupboards are brimming with food you're trying to get rid of!

TIME/MONEY SAVER #3: PREP AHEAD

Now that you have everything you need for the week, go the extra mile and prepare some of your meals ahead to save effort all week long. Get out your cutting board to chop and portion vegetables and most fruits (hold off on apples and berries). Place them in sealed containers—one for snacks or lunch boxes for the week, one for salads, and one ready to sauté, grill, or roast. Make your own tuna, chicken, or egg salad. Put together an entire week's worth of lunches and refrigerate. Freeze smoothie bags with all the ingredients ready to go and thaw the night before in the refrigerator. If you're grilling on the weekend, make extra vegetables to add to quesadillas, salads, wraps, or pizza. You'd be amazed how much advanced prep you can get done in the thirty minutes after you get back from the store. You won't have to go through it all again every weeknight, and cooking suddenly becomes more delightful.

TIME/MONEY SAVER #4: GET COOKING

Nothing teaches you how to cook better than just rolling up your sleeves and trying it out. Choose recipes that don't take much time to prepare, such as fish, tacos, and one-pot "chop and drop" recipes.

Slow cookers are great for meals that cook themselves. I also like casseroles you can assemble over the weekend and bake on a busy weeknight—freeing up your time for a quick workout. If you're feeling adventurous, try out a friend's pressure cooker. Today's models are easy to use and get a pot roast and potato dinner on the table in record time.

After dinner each night, refrigerate or freeze room-temperature foods. This may be a good time to adjust your menu if you have more leftover food than expected. When the next weekend rolls around, you'll repeat these steps and start your meal plan all over with the food you have on hand. If you're like most people, you probably have not used everything you thought you would. You may have one or two days' worth of meals and you might be worried that your fresh food will go bad—not if you use it or freeze it! Challenge yourself to find a good use for that food (and next time, buy less). You should notice savings at the grocery store, less food in the trash, and more time on your hands if you keep practicing these tips.

TIME/MONEY SAVER #5: MAKE YOUR KITCHEN WORK FOR YOU

As you get the hang of these food routines, there's one more thing you can do—make your kitchen a place you actually *want* to cook—or at least a place where you can work more efficiently because you can find everything. Refresh your kitchen without the pricey budget of a remodel with these four simple steps—remove, clean, toss, and organize. Give yourself a good half day and get all corners of your kitchen done, including refrigerator, freezer, pantry, cupboards, drawers, and countertops.

....

REMOVE—Take everything out. If it's repulsive or looks like a chemistry experiment, just go ahead and toss it now. But don't dawdle with this step. The goal here is to get everything in plain sight at once and make the next steps more efficient.

....

CLEAN—Wipe down all surfaces with a solution of warm water and a few drops of dish soap. Disinfect with a 50/50 solution of white vinegar and water or use a gallon of water and ½ cup bleach for a more powerful job. Follow up with a wipe down of just plain water.

....

TOSS—While all your surfaces are drying, it's time to toss! Check all foods, vitamins, supplements, herbs, and spices for dates. Toss everything that's expired. Set a timer to encourage yourself to work fast. You could spend all day overthinking and searching for a reason why you need to keep both the toaster oven and the toaster, or why you just can't let go of a few coffee mugs even though you can't close your cabinet doors. If you don't use it at least once a week, why is it taking up space? If you really can't part with it, try putting it in a box and storing it away with your holiday decorations. If you see that box the next time the holidays roll around and you didn't miss anything, drive that stuff to Goodwill immediately!

....

ORGANIZE—Wipe down everything you're keeping with a damp cloth before putting it back in its ideal place. Group foods that go together, like condiments, dried goods, and canned foods you usually use in the same dish. My tomato paste is near diced tomatoes and tomato sauce, chickpeas near tuna fish, and black beans near chilis, corn, and hot sauce. Use the first in, first out method to avoid food waste. The foods you want to use first should be in the front of the refrigerator, freezer, and pantry. While you're organizing, it's a great time to write down meal ideas to use up some of the food you didn't want to toss, and take note if you are overstocked with any food. You may also note if you need to replace storage containers or purchase anything else that would really help you work swiftly in the kitchen. Check your cleaning supplies. Before you finish, place a large clear bowl of fresh fruit on your kitchen table or countertop for easy snacking and a beautiful centerpiece.

There are many more resources online for how to create a kitchen that works for you. Start with these four steps and advance your skills from there. When you put in the effort to clean and organize your kitchen, your sense of accomplishment gives you just that little spiral up boost of energy you need to look forward to using it. And when it gets disheveled every week (or every day), it's a lot easier to beautify with a few quick steps.

Making the Most of Fitness

I focused most of my time- and money-saving tips on food, but I don't want to leave you in the dark with fitness. The most magical way of saving time and money on fitness is by choosing free or inexpensive activities and building movement into your day. If your exercise isn't happening—why? What do you need that you don't already have? If time continues to be a problem, consider the shortest workout possible you could do at home, work, or wherever you are. Revisit the ideas from the fitness chapter, Chapter 3, especially overcoming the "I don't have time" roadblock, and check your journal notes if you need inspiration.

A week of successful movement for a time-starved person may look something like this:

MONDAY: Seven-minute full body workout (free app)

TUESDAY: Fifteen-minute power walk with coworker to grab lunch. Plus walk home from work (free).

WEDNESDAY: Yoga class, one hour, plus twenty minutes' drive time

THURSDAY: Twenty-minute DVD at home while dinner cooks in oven

FRIDAY: Thirty-minute jog before work (free)

SATURDAY: Meet a girlfriend to run errands on foot. Coffee together after (free, if she buys the coffee).

SUNDAY: Blast upbeat music and boogie while doing chores with family (free)

Track Your Progress Daily

It can be helpful to have a sense each day that you are accomplishing something. I encourage you to check in with yourself daily using low-tech, paper-based tools, such as reflective journaling or a simple body kindness checklist. You should be able to tell in a minute's review how you are progressing at goals that are important to you.

Take a few minutes and make a list of body kindness actions. Here are some examples of items you could include on your list:

Did I enjoy my meals?

Did I eat mindfully, in a way that feels good?

Are my food choices energizing me?

Did I build balanced plates?

Did I "surf the urge" to eat my feelings?

Did I move my body and have some fun with it?

Did I sleep enough?

Have I been kind to others and myself?

Did I shut down technology by 8 p.m.?

Did I laugh and smile today?

Did I drink enough water?

Did I cope with stress and negative emotions in helpful ways?

Overall, do I feel satisfied with my self-care today?

You can also boost your awareness of progress by journaling each day about your highs and lows, which can also bring attention to how you're speaking to yourself. If you make a mistake or choose something that isn't in line with your goals, it's OK. With mindfulness, you recognize that the choice you made was not the best, accept it, and go on to choose the next meaningful option to spiral up. Start small, be realistic, and forgive yourself easily when you get sidetracked. The important thing is to come back to the routine you planned because it's based on what is most important to you.

An evening reflection is a good time to set intentions for the next day. When you rise each morning, you can check in. Ask yourself: How do I feel? How committed am I to today's goals? You might notice you are tired or feeling low in energy, despite your commitment to body kindness. In my experience, the top reason people don't develop the health habits they want is because their pessimism is too high and grit is too low. If you don't fully respect the process of behavior change, you see difficulty as failure and a sign to quit. Your thought bullies are in full force and you don't use your tools to disengage them. Don't quit, grow your grit. Angela Duckworth, author of *Grit: The Power of Passion and Perseverance*, says anyone can improve their grit by consistently challenging themselves—see it as "practice," enjoy your effort regardless of the outcome, and be courageous. Do what's important even if you're afraid, and welcome frustration as a sign of progress—you're doing something to change and it's supposed to be difficult.

. . . .

BODY KINDNESS REFLECTION: Spend fifteen minutes thinking about what it is going to take for you to make over your schedule. Think about how important it is for you to be able to follow your body kindness blueprint. If any negative thoughts arise, just notice them and write down why you are committed to finding the time you need for yourself.

. . . .

> "A goal without a plan is just a wish."
> —Antoine de Saint-Exupéry

Chapter 10

Befriend Yourself

The Beautiful Power of Self-Compassion

Philosophy

The most important relationship in your life is the one you have with yourself. Treating this relationship with loving care, as if you were your best friend, will accelerate your progress toward your goals. Whether you want to do better at honoring your personal values or you need to call a truce in an all-out war against yourself, body kindness offers a framework for transforming your relationship with you. Befriending yourself is the next important step you will take toward a healthier and happier life. The benefits of a strong bond between your heart, body, and mind include feeling more positive emotions, easier decision-making, and trusting in the process of behavior change, even in the midst of setbacks. Respecting who you already are will help you become the person you want to be.

BODY KINDNESS PILLARS
Making Peace with Yourself

LOVE: Practicing self-compassion and self-acceptance are acts of love. When you make mistakes, get stuck, or when you're just not feeling the love from yourself, try to be more understanding, kind, and respectful.

CONNECT: Open up a dialogue with yourself to build an alliance. Communicate how you're doing and what needs your attention in the present moment, as you work on changing your habits.

CARE: Be good to yourself no matter what. Trust that you will be gentle, honest, and fair in your caregiving, like the way you would treat a child who needs your nurturing.

Why You Must Befriend Yourself

Imagine being stuck in a car with someone you don't particularly like—maybe a coworker or not-so-friendly neighbor. But there you are sitting next to each other. Unpleasant! Now imagine that car ride never ends. Excruciating! You're going to be with yourself for a very long time. It's a good idea to find a way to get along and maybe enjoy the ride.

I have a saying with clients—"You can't hate yourself healthy." No matter how much you berate yourself for not being the way you think you should be, you won't truly create the better life you desire unless you start from a place of love. But loving yourself is not easy for everyone, especially when you feel inadequate or you're grappling with shame. As you begin to work through habit changes, body kindness can be particularly challenging when you don't effortlessly do what you set out to do. Look what you have accomplished. You've done all this work thinking about what you really want, identified your values, brainstormed goals, and created a plan to follow. You may have gotten further than you ever have before, and yet you have no guarantee that you

Spiral Up

Imagine you had a do-over. The older, wiser you could return to any point in your life and share inspirations, lessons, or regrets. Take fifteen minutes and write in your journal. Think of different ages and stages of your life so far. What would you say to yourself at ten years old, your high school self, your college self? What do your words tell you about acceptance and self-compassion? What do you want your future, wiser self to say to you right now to help you on this body kindness journey?

will achieve your goals in the long run. That's scary! It's perfectly normal to feel uncertainty and self-doubt. When you're straddling the crossroads of change, you just want to shed your current life and run away from all the things you dislike now and—BAM! Be that new and improved person. But there are no shortcuts. **The magic of transformation is in the process—the highs, the lows, the failures and triumphs.** You become who you want to be by working with the person you already are—collaboratively taking actions to accomplish goals, learning and growing with each moment. Until one day you suddenly realize you're there. Let me tell you this. Your fear is real. Your doubts are real. Some days will be hard. Self-improvement is some of the toughest work anyone can do. We all struggle, even when our lives are much better than before! No matter what lies ahead, you have never been more prepared than you are in this moment. You have never been better set up for long-term success.

Now is when you need to show up for yourself more than ever. Don't reject yourself. Befriend yourself. Start by letting "the good" sink in. Allow yourself to acknowledge any small steps that you've taken since you started reading this book. Celebrate the "good enough" effort you have made, even if you want to do more. Remember that you have what you need to succeed—both the desire and resources to make changes stick. You just need to be patient with yourself and keep practicing. *Act. Repeat. Mess up. Reflect. Act again.* That's the true path of forming new habits. It's not a straight line forward. It's a windy, messy, crooked, challenging, and sometimes confusing road. Walk toward difficulty fearlessly. It's like strength training for your brain. It doesn't matter if you mess up; all that matters is you are putting forth effort. When you are trying, you are changing. You will be much more encouraged to keep trying when you are coaching yourself, "Keep going, friend. You got this."

Practices to Help You Befriend Yourself

These body kindness essentials will help you become better at being good to yourself, and you might notice how using previous skills—like the PACT (Presence, Acceptance, Choice, Take action) approach—involves use of these practices.

MINDFULNESS—Paying attention to whatever is happening in the present moment, without judgment whenever possible.

SELF-COMPASSION—Valuing your well-being and responding to challenges with kindness and support.

SELF-ACCEPTANCE—Acknowledging the good, the bad, and the ugly of what it means to be human, and giving yourself permission to just be who you are.

GRATITUDE—Cultivating a mindful appreciation for life's gifts.

AFFIRMATIONS—Reinforcing self-care through positive statements that reflect loving-kindness toward yourself.

My hunch is you're already making progress in a few of these areas, or maybe you can see them reflected in your values, goals, and body kindness blueprint. For example, you've likely practiced mindfulness ("I notice these thoughts and feelings."), acceptance ("The thoughts and feelings are allowed to be here."), and self-compassion ("This is difficult, but I will be OK"). While each of these skills is uniquely important on its own, they are somewhat of a package deal. You're more likely to improve a little in all of these areas by practicing one of them. By committing to an honest and collaborative relationship with yourself, you are connecting with your inner caregiver and building a strong foundation for all of your body kindness goals.

Mindfulness Comes First

Mindfulness underscores all the other body kindness essentials for befriending yourself, and it's the first step when you're using the PACT approach for decision-making (Presence). Even with the best of intentions, taking care of ourselves, our work, our homes, and our loved ones can be all-consuming. It can feel like you're always running around, frantically trying to check items off your to-do list, and there are never enough hours in the day. When things go wrong, which they inevitably do, that's when we're likely to hear one of the thought bullies chime in with self-criticism. We often don't notice our own pain or suffering when it's happening. **Mindfulness opens the door to a different way of handling life when it feels like you're your own worst enemy.**

By paying attention in the present moment, without making any judgments regarding the things you experience and observe, you are strengthening your body and mind's natural ability to respond to stress. And just like any form of exercise, the more you do it, the better the results you can achieve. You might recall other activities from previous chapters that seem a lot like mindfulness; that's not an accident. The state of observing rather than judging keeps your mind open to rational thinking about the next choice you want to make. The more you practice this gentle attention in any aspect of life, the more upward spirals you'll experience.

Developing a simple mindfulness-based meditative practice can help you center yourself, decrease stress, and gain clarity before reacting to a situation. This might be as simple as deep breathing or a daily ritual where you spend five minutes alone, noticing what you see, hear, and feel in a more mindful way. Taking time to truly be present allows us to reconnect with our bodies and give our overactive brains a rest. Mindfulness can also help you become more aware of how you speak to and about yourself. Too often we say hurtful things without even thinking. What's one thing you said to yourself that you would not want your friend or partner to know you said because it's too painful? It's not hard to come up with a handful of criticism. We all do it. Disparaging ourselves isn't helpful or motivating, and it can be harmful, with lasting consequences to our self-esteem and self-worth. So when you notice a thought bully seeping out into conversation, try to respond with compassion. But first, try the body scan as a way to become friendlier with yourself and build mindfulness at the same time.

BUILDING SELF-COMPASSION

When mindfulness helps us notice our suffering, self-compassion comes in with a helpful response that lifts our mood and inspires us to keep going. Many people believe they need to be hard on themselves in order to change. Not only is that untrue—it has the opposite of the intended effect. Beating yourself up actually makes you less likely to stay committed to any goal you set for yourself. But when self-compassion is high, you are much more likely to take responsibility for your actions and do something to change your direction.

Self-compassion is about treating yourself with kindness and respect throughout normal, everyday life— when you're not feeling your best, when your thought bullies are coming in for the attack, or when, inevitably, mistakes and challenges occur. You

YOUR BODY SCAN
BOOST AWARENESS AND MINDFULNESS

FROM ACHES AND pains to muscular tension, nervous energy, and restlessness, our bodies are constantly communicating with us. Our muscles tell us to take it slow or stretch it out, and our nervous systems let us know that something is important or needs our attention. Developing an awareness of all these signals starts with taking time to check in with your body. Try the following body scan exercise. Body scans work best when you are open to connecting to your body. If you feel uncomfortable, remember this is a neutral observation and try to keep it a judgment-free zone.

1. Lie down or sit in a comfortable position, preferably somewhere quiet, without interruptions.

4. You can start from head to toe or vice versa. I usually start from my toes and work my way up.

2. Begin by noticing how your chest and belly move up and down with each inhalation and exhalation.

3. Do this for several breaths, and then begin to expand your awareness to include the rest of your body.

5. Bring your attention to each part of your body, progressing through each toe, to the ball of your foot, up to your arches and heels. Take your time.

6. The key is not to try and adjust or fix anything. Just settle into the awareness of all the sensations. Notice if each body part is cold or warm, tense or relaxed, restless or calm. If you move gently, bring your awareness to it.

8. We all hold our stress in different locations throughout the body. When you come to your shoulders and neck, you may feel tightness, heaviness, or even pain. Sometimes just the recognition of these sensations helps relax and soothe these areas.

7. As you work your way up, focus on your muscles, joints, and bones. Is anything sore, tense, or relaxed? How does your skin feel? Is your heart racing or beating normally?

9. Continue with your jaw, mouth, and tongue. Are you clenching muscles in your face? Are you furrowing your brow? Let those sensations be known and allow them to melt away.

10. Finish at the top of your head and allow yourself to rest in that fully aware and connected state. I try to allow ten to twenty minutes to complete the entire scan, but even a quick five-minute body scan will help strengthen your mind-body connection. The practice of observing will help you be more mindful next time you're all worked up.

Spiral Up
FINDING YOUR
SELF-COMPASSION

Get a sense of how good you are at self-compassion by reflecting on times in your life when you're more likely to be gentle with yourself and when you're more likely to be harsh and unforgiving. Open your journal and complete these phrases.

Moments of strength: I tend to have the most self-compassion when _____ .

Moments of difficulty: I struggle with self-compassion when _____ .

If I could practice having more self-compassion, I would do more _____ when I am _____ . I would do less _____ when I am _____ .

Think about how your responses could help you create a better life and move you closer to your health goals. How would your inner caregiver help you through times when self-compassion is difficult?

might say something like "This is really difficult. I'm not alone in feeling this way. What can I do for myself right now in this moment?" People with self-compassion skills have a higher sense of self-worth, have better body image, and are intrinsically motivated to prioritize self-care. Self-compassion is strongly linked to lower rates of depression, anxiety, perfectionism, and ruminating on negative thoughts. These people are also less likely to compare themselves to others, which is generally unhelpful (remember "compare and despair"), and more likely to be optimistic, curious, grateful, and satisfied with life. These skills aren't

necessarily something we're all born with, and self-compassion is certainly not something our competitive world is begging to teach us. Thankfully, you can develop these skills, because they are vitally essential to body kindness.

Using self-compassion, you can turn mindfulness into action. Think about one time recently when you noticed downward spiraling and you jumped in to reverse it. You successfully used mindfulness and self-compassion to get there! And every time you spiral up, you strengthen your mindfulness and self-compassion skills. In order to reverse your downward spirals, you need to be aware that they're happening and you need to feel a desire to respond with kindness. For example, my friend Pam shared with me the story of how a heavy dose of self-compassion helped transform her life:

I spent almost ten years berating myself in a million different ways for not being a happy homemaker. Every time the kitchen floor was sticky, I spiraled down and blamed myself for not being able to handle everything. I remember sitting with my sons at the park and looking at all the other moms, thinking their lives looked so simple and happy. I stopped doing most of the things I cared about, hoping that if I was less busy I could keep up. But the simpler my life became, the more empty I felt inside and the more mistakes I seemed to make. Eventually the voice in my head became so defeating that I started to believe I would just have to suffer through the next eighteen years until there were fewer messes to clean up. I feel so sad now, thinking about the way I treated myself. I wasn't incompetent! I was human. I spent all my time and energy taking care of other people, and I did absolutely nothing to take care of myself. Finally, when my therapist encouraged me to start a journal, it uncovered the creative part of my spirit that had been buried underneath all those negative words. Something came back to life and now I am healthier than I have ever been. My personal mantra these days is "perfection is not the goal," and I use it a lot! Everyone has gifts and talents that bring goodness to the world, and mine have nothing to do with a clean house. It's not a coincidence that my marriage, my career, and my kids are all happier now that I started treating myself with the same compassion and respect I had always given to everyone else.

The best way I've found to teach clients self-compassion is to rehearse how they would respond to their struggle if they were hearing it from a friend. First, think about a friend you love. Imagine her struggling in some way. How would you respond to her in this situation? What would you do and say, and what is your tone of voice like when you talk to her? Practice using that same tone of voice and those caring gestures the next time you start to feel the voice of discouragement seep into your own thoughts. **When your inner bullies get too noisy, catch yourself in the act and stick up for yourself! "Oh my gosh, will you give this hardworking woman a break?** Look at all she's juggling. She needs your encouragement, not judgment! If you don't have anything nice to say, then leave her alone!" The following is an excerpt from a letter one client wrote to her younger self, as a reminder of the self-compassion she is trying to create in her older, wiser years.

Dear Maggie,

I could write you a novel about all of the things I wish you had done differently based on the things I know now. I would have told you to study abroad, to study a field you liked in college, to learn a second language, to drink less Diet Coke, to be less self-conscious, to invest more time in understanding what makes you happy, to never go on a fad diet (or better yet, to never worry about food), to enjoy little moments more, to floss your teeth, and to enjoy your curly hair while it lasted.

But, the truth is, I would tell myself all of this, and then ask myself to not listen to older me. Because all of those missteps and awkward experiences somehow worked together to create someone that I'm happy to know now. There are wild moments of imperfection in my life and a million things that probably should have or could have been done differently on the micro level, but on the macro level, it is all working out OK.

So, the bottom line is, I would tell myself to enjoy the ride and to not worry too much about the "mistakes" because, in the long run, it all works out.

This is the way I need to treat myself now. I need to give myself permission to make mistakes—even be grateful for them because they are part of what makes me complete.

Love, Maggie

Prominent self-compassion researcher and author Kristin Neff says there are three elements of self-compassion. We have covered two—mindfulness and self-kindness. The third is common

humanity. I find it most effective for relieving me of self-criticism, such as "I'm not the only one going through this crap!" It's such a relief to know I'm not alone. We all suffer and we can persevere. When I hear this "I'm messed up" talk from clients, I often respond, "Sorry, but there's nothing special about you." And then I tell them a story of someone who dealt with a similar problem. Knowing other people struggle—even really successful people—leads to upward spirals. I was listening to a panel discussion of "power moms," including NASA astronaut Cady Coleman, who spent six months at the international space station—outer space! When asked about regrets, they said the all-too-familiar "I wish I worked less, I wish I was more present when I was with my family and not distracted by work and my own thoughts, and I wish I managed my time better." It made my day because how they feel is exactly how I feel most of the time. It inspired me to think of our shared humanity the next time I wanted to put myself in "mom jail" for not giving my all.

If you would like to test how self-compassionate you are, take Neff's free online quiz at SelfCompassion.org and use her tools to help you bring more self-compassion into your life.

LOVING-KINDNESS MEDITATION

The loving-kindness meditation has been used for years and has many forms.

Researchers have studied its effectiveness in well-being, including improving self-compassion. You can find plenty of versions of loving-kindness meditation (also known as metta) online. While there are many ways to practice loving-kindness meditation, a simplified form is to repeat silently, while you are comfortably seated, phrases like the following for a period of time: *"May I feel safe. May I feel happy. May I feel healthy and strong. May I live with ease."* and keep returning to these thoughts when your mind wanders.

Loving-kindness meditation has been shown to change the structure and function of the brain and is a highly effective way to fortify compassion and acceptance of yourself and others. You can direct similar thoughts toward loved ones, strangers, or people with whom there is conflict or tension. Some of my clients prefer to start their meditation toward someone else for a few minutes before sending themselves loving-kindness.

I cannot understate the importance of self-compassion in befriending yourself. In my experience, it's the last thing clients want to do. They practically squirm in their chairs at the thought of sending themselves good vibes and warm feelings, particularly when they're disappointed about something. I can't tell you how often I've heard the words "I love myself; that's not the problem." But it is the problem. They say they love themselves, but in certain situations they don't treat themselves like they do. They get caught up in feelings of anger and disgust, and before you know it they start to get impatient and give up. We don't tell our loved ones they are worthless. We don't tell them to quit striving for their goals. Most of us would never even consider calling another person fat, ugly, or lazy. But we don't think twice about saying that to ourselves. It's time we started providing the same compassionate, encouraging support to ourselves that we provide to other people.

FAILURE IS A GIFT

Let's acknowledge that failure happens to everyone. When I make progress toward a goal, my joy at the achievement is immediately followed by, "Oh my God, you could lose it all." I scold myself that I'm not doing enough to succeed and I'll soon be labeled with the scarlet letter "F." I tell myself that I have no idea what I'm doing (not true) and that the people I love the most are going to suffer from my inadequacies (not true). Any time we are faced with difficulty, fear and its evil cohorts—judgment, criticism, and perfectionism—will inevitably rear their ugly heads. The beauty is that you can choose to say "bring it on" to all that failure can teach you. When you're not criticizing yourself, you can befriend yourself instead and be there to pick yourself up when you fall.

In her book *Fail, Fail Again, Fail Better*, Pema Chödrön says that failure is actually the most direct way to become a more complete, loving, and fulfilled human being. If we want to live a rewarding life, we need to stay open, take risks, and be present when things don't work out. When you appreciate failure for what it really is—an opportunity to teach you something, to give you feedback, to provide information—you can make good use of your new knowledge to make your next choices.

Failure can be any situation that we feel is not a success or where the outcome doesn't match our expectation. This might be something as simple as lashing out in anger at someone you love or as painful as the end of an important relationship. Most of us tend to add up our failures and hold them up as evidence of our own limited self-worth—especially when we don't complete meaningful goals. I'm sure everyone reading this book has started an exercise plan they never finished or a diet they weren't able to maintain. Some failures can be particularly embarrassing, but this is often where the most opportunity for reflection and growth lies. I have a lot of respect for Bernie Salazar, my dear friend who was the runner-up on the TV show *The Biggest Loser*, season five. (He lost the most weight of any contestant sent home, "winning" the second place prize.) Eight years later, Bernie talked candidly about his struggle to find his true health after the spotlight faded. When he realized the expectations he developed through intense exercise

and strict eating were not sustainable, Bernie penned the "Loser Letter" and read it to me during one of my Body Kindness podcasts. He intended to help the contestants from the most recent season, but Bernie soon realized he was talking to himself and anyone else struggling to make sense of failure in behavior change. He offered three pieces of advice in his letter. He encouraged people to take time to get to their core issues, working with professionals and with support from people they trust. He suggested people evaluate relationships, being open to new ones and prepared for old ones to fade away. His third tip meant the most to me because it represents the root cause of his failure and the solution for his success.

"Redefine what health means to you— Through hard work and careful self-reflection, I have moved past the rhetoric and actually understand and value what I was just sort of spouting off back when I first left the show. Knowing that working out three to six hours a day isn't realistic or that counting every single calorie you consume will eventually get old, how will you choose to define "health," so that the definition contributes to your well-being rather than stands for something you are in constant fear of not living up to? Redefining what "health" means to you will help you face the inevitable barriers you will encounter along your journey. Most important, having a clear definition will provide room for honest

self-reflection, complete self-care, true body kindness, and lasting happiness."

Bernie didn't have a workable definition of health when he started making behavior changes. He learned his "Loser Lessons" the hard way, by fighting his body as he tried to hang on to unrealistic ideals and behaviors. But the failure he felt is not likely explained solely by the fault of his own habits. Recent research points to clinical data demonstrating that the body appears to fight back after weight loss by slowing metabolism so that despite eating fewer calories and feeling hungry, the body hangs on to pounds or adds them back on. It's an evolutionary mechanism and not about willpower. We aren't supposed to work *against* our bodies. We need to broaden the idea of what health really means for individuals, families, communities, and the human race. We have to ask how ethical it is to subject people to diets if the goal of health care is do no harm—because diets, by and large, are harmful.

By looking inward and sharing this experience with other people, Bernie continues to touch more lives than he ever anticipated, even though his outcome doesn't match the traditional (and unrealistic) image of a happily-ever-after "success story." The big question for you is: When you notice a failure, how will you forgive and move on?

When you make mistakes big or small, you need to be able to remember your values—what you care about and

why—so you can move forward. One choice, the very next choice you make, can get you spiraling up in the right direction again. Staying fused to feelings of guilt, shame, or judgment keeps you holding on to events of the past. You can't go back and change them, but you can let go and move forward. Your ability to recognize mistakes, learn, plan for the next time, and continue on your journey will help determine how quickly you change and how you feel throughout the process. Journaling and creativity are both powerful tools for moving past failure to forgiveness. If you're feeling stuck in a negative emotional space, I encourage you to record all your feelings, without judgment, and then push yourself a little harder, digging deeper to tell the true story that is below the surface.

Self-Acceptance

Now it's time to apply the second part of the PACT strategy (Acceptance) to your personal relationship with yourself. I want to be clear—*acceptance* is not *apathy*. It is not giving up. It's not ignoring your goals and refusing self-improvement. Self-acceptance means acknowledging what you do and don't have the power to change, so you can move forward and become the person you want to be.

My sister-in-law Hayley is a busy, confident mother of two young girls, and few people would imagine all of the things she has learned to accept over the years to become the happy, loving person she is today. Since elementary school, Hayley's struggles with dyslexia and ADD have affected her relationships and self-image. Not only was she teased for being different, but at one point she had unexplainable physical symptoms and a terrible rumor was circulating that she had AIDS. You don't have to know much about preteen girls to imagine what this did to her self-esteem and her social life.

No matter what her parents and teachers said, Hayley couldn't see her worthiness through all her academic and social struggles. She became withdrawn and lost interest in activities she had previously enjoyed. But then one day, someone introduced Hayley to the beautiful world of Japanese origami art. "I couldn't believe all the creations you could do with paper. I would sit for hours and pass the time making origami birds, angelfish, and frogs. Through origami, I discovered I liked to draw and design. To my surprise, I had skills other people didn't. I was creative! It was such a relief to learn that I was more than my disability." And being able to share that creative part of herself with others opened up a world of service and self-expression where Hayley continues to thrive.

Whether she is crafting with her kids or running a PTA fund-raiser, Hayley's ability to accept her challenges comes from finding ways to focus on her strengths.

"I feel secure and loved. I contribute to something that matters. My confidence grows. I get a certain energy when I'm doing something like this, and I feel good about myself in every way. Suddenly criticisms about my brain or body don't matter to me." When she embraces her natural abilities and affirms her value in other areas of her life, it strengthens her confidence for situations she may have struggled with in the past. "Certain things will always be more challenging for me—like following a simple recipe. It can get really frustrating. But I've learned to accept, and even embrace, my barriers, which has helped me be more self-compassionate and ultimately more successful."

What are you really good at? Spend more time celebrating and connecting with that part of yourself. Doing so will make it much easier to accept and embrace parts of yourself that are holding you back and weighing you down.

MAKING PEACE WITH YOUR BODY

The very first thought that came to mind when I sat down to write about body acceptance was "Rebecca, who do you think you are? You are the last person in the world who should be telling people how to make peace with their appearance." Thankfully I practice self-compassion and have the flexibility to tolerate that crappy thought. My truth is I'm better qualified *because* I've suffered from poor body image for

Spiral Up

Write yourself some love notes. Use the power of community and ask your friends on social media to share their words of wisdom, or look back on cards that have been given to you in the past, then print/copy and cut/paste on note cards to keep those love notes around for a time when you might need them. Here are few quick ones my friends shared when I asked for words of wisdom and self-love:

★ *Think about being pretty*. Be pretty kind. Pretty funny. Pretty smart and pretty strong!

★ *It's OK to be scared*. You're about to do something that matters.

★ *Pay yourself first*—time alone, hobbies, travel, etc.—and everyone else can have what's left over.

★ *"Be patient* toward all that is unsolved in your heart and try to love the questions themselves." —Rainer Maria Rilke

★ *She believed* she could, so she did.

★ *Perfection* is SO overrated. It's sterile and unfriendly.

★ *Be kind*. Be truly, really kind to yourself and to others.

★ *Be musical*. Make yourself an "All About Me" playlist to get you pumped up about how amazing it is to be YOU. Lady Gaga's "Born This Way" and Pharrell's "Happy" are fun starting tunes.

years. I have felt the shame of not feeling worthy of love and friendship or a bikini. As young, single adults, my friend Lindsay and I would pinch our belly rolls to make a pair of lips that could "speak" and say denigrating things about their owners (ourselves). While we chalked this up to being silly, I now realize we weren't exactly expressing self-acceptance. We were beating ourselves up and laughing about it. It's not like we were alone in body bashing. In fact, an overwhelming majority of women have an "I hate my body" moment every single day. Nearly half of three- to six-year-olds are afraid of being fat. The average age girls start their first diet is eight years old. We carry these scars with us, and only a few of us

HOW MUCH DO YOU APPRECIATE YOUR BODY?
Take this quiz to find out.

Tylka Body Appreciation Scale*
For each item, the following response scale should be used: 1 = Never, 2 = Seldom, 3 = Sometimes, 4 = Often, 5 = Always.

1   I respect my body.

2   I feel good about my body.

3   I feel that my body has at least some good qualities.

4   I take a positive attitude toward my body.

5   I am attentive to my body's needs.

6   I feel love for my body.

7   I appreciate the different and unique characteristics of my body.

8   My behavior reveals my positive attitude toward my body; for example, I hold my head high and smile.

9   I am comfortable in my body.

10   I feel like I am beautiful even if I am different from media images of attractive people (e.g., models, actresses/actors).

Scoring Procedure: Calculate the average for your responses.

The closer your score is to 5, the more appreciation you have for your body. Review any low scores, journal about why you have trouble with those areas, and generate ideas for growing your body appreciation.

* Copyright Dr. Tracy Tylka

are lucky enough to not be bothered by poor body image. The undeniable truth is that we are subject to stigma about our weight, we internalize it, and we either fight it or we use stigma to fight ourselves.

One of my clients wrote, "I've been cursed with a pear-shaped body. Horrible genetics. I've got very narrow shoulders, wide hips that look as though I'm about to drop twin sumo wrestlers, and short legs. I feel like I've tried every diet and workout, but nothing seems to help. And just being in the gym around well-sculpted bodies, knowing that I could never look anything like them, is soul crushing. I just want to escape this body sometimes [sad face]."

Another client, Robby, said she needed to shift her mindset from blaming herself, in order to finally accept her body and truly take care of it. "I have struggled with my weight, shape, and my size for years. When I thought it was all genetics, I was angry with what nature gave me. When I realized it wasn't all genetics, I got mad at my circumstances and environment when things didn't go right. I learned that when we struggle with something, it's usually because we're trying to avoid accepting things as they are. But when I finally stopped trying to blame everything, including myself, I began to reconcile the dissonance between what I believed, how I acted, and what I looked like. Struggling against myself wasn't making things easier; guilt and blame were just distracting me from the one action that would actually put me on the path of the body and life I wanted. I needed to make peace with the past and learn how to love myself (my *whole* self, including the 'fat suit') as I was and as I am. The practice of finding that peace helped me discover the wealth of love and admiration that I had for myself. I can now recognize when I'm beating myself up, and I'm strong enough (and vocal enough) to defend/protect my imperfectly wonderful self

from a society that thrives on self-loathing. I know I'm healthy and strong, and I think one small thing I can do to help change society is to accept myself. Maybe if we all accept ourselves, society will become more accepting of diverse bodies."

I know many women who don't look like "the ideal" body, and they are healthy and strong. They are spin instructors, Ironman athletes, personal trainers, working professionals, moms, teachers, and graduate students. Yet I know others who could be healthier and stronger if they just made peace with their bodies and did the best they could, despite the shortcomings of our judgmental society.

Self-acceptance is a lifelong journey. You'll need time and patience to adjust to being a person who practices body kindness, and who doesn't diet. The one habit that corresponds most closely with us being satisfied with our lives overall—self-acceptance—is often the one we practice least. When we're self-accepting, we're able to embrace *all* facets of ourselves—not just the parts we love. Authenticity is essential to befriending yourself with a whole and open heart. You do not need to fake body positivity that is not there. You don't have to say, "I love every curve, wrinkle, dimple, and flaw of me" if you don't actually feel it. You can be body positive while still being a truthful human being. While it's OK to acknowledge weaknesses and insecurities, true self-acceptance is unconditional. By bringing your beliefs

Spiral Up
YOUR BODY KINDNESS BALANCE SHEET

EACH TIME YOU:	BALANCE IT WITH:
Insult yourself	A compliment
Spend too much time at the mirror	Hang a towel over it for a few days or cover it up with gorgeous wrapping paper—a present to yourself.
Find that something doesn't fit	Donate it and buy a new, comfortable outfit.
Receive a compliment	Remember that "Thank you" is a complete sentence, and there's no need to disagree with someone else's compliment.
Compare yourself to others	Say out loud five things you are good at.
Make a mistake	Say "I forgive you."
Hide from a camera	Take a selfie with someone you love, and smile!

into the light, you can see them for what they are and still choose the path that moves you forward to create a better life. And it includes "loving" (or at least respecting) the imperfect parts of yourself in a way that is personally meaningful.

Beloved author Anne Lamott could be considered a self-acceptance expert. On social media and in her books, Lamott candidly shares her own lifelong battle with food and body image, and her eventual reconciliation that the path to healthier living must be paved in profound self-love, kindness, and grace. She tells us, "Unfortunately, it's yet another inside job. If you are not OK with yourself at 185 [pounds], you will not be OK at 150, or even 135. The self-respect and peace of mind you long for is not out there. It's within. I hate that. I resent that more than I can say. But it's true. Maybe some of us can try to eat a bit less and walk a bit more, and make sure to wear pants that do not hurt our thighs or our feelings."

The real message is that to have a more fulfilling life, you need body acceptance, not weight loss. While social media and mainstream culture want us to believe there is a single mold we should all fit into, one of the greatest parts of being human is that each one of us is unique. For many of us, it can take a lifetime to separate our own inner voice from the noise of the crowd. But when we learn to respect and appreciate the differences and diversity of human nature, the next step is to expand that acceptance to include ourselves.

Repeat after me: "My body is not the problem." Body image has little to do with your actual size or shape. It's all about your personal perception of your body. A healthy body image occurs when a person is able to accept, appreciate, and respect their body. Notice that this definition makes no mention of weight, and therefore honors the fact that people naturally come in different shapes and sizes.

If the body appreciation quiz reveals that you're unhappy about your body, try to dig a little deeper and connect with the value that is reflected in your discomfort. Do you personally want to feel better in your own body, or is it because you feel others expect you to look a certain way? What does healthy and beautiful look like to you? It's exhausting to live by other people's—or marketing companies'—standards. But remember, just because you have a thought doesn't mean it's a fact—often just the opposite! Remember, if your thought doesn't help you create a better life, then it's not useful to you. *Next, please.* As you integrate more self-compassion and self-empathy into your daily life, you'll begin to catch yourself when the inner bully gets started, and you can make a choice to redirect the conversation toward a more positive dialogue.

Now let's apply the PACT process to your goals for befriending and body appreciation:

PRESENCE: For instance, you're looking at photos someone just posted online—"Wow. Look at all my chins in that photograph. Everyone around me looks great. I look frumpy, tired, and unhappy." *Screech!* Time to put the brakes on. Ask yourself what useful information you can glean from noticing that thought.

ACCEPTANCE: Try to forget about the rest of it and focus on whatever part is helpful. Noticing that you don't look happy and also noticing the way you just insulted yourself speaks to a value conflict. "I want to be a person who speaks gently to myself."

CHOICE: You had a negative thought about your chin and the way you look. No big deal. Now decide what you want to do (if anything) to change the situation. Will you ask your friend to delete the photo? Or spend a few moments replacing your inner dialogue with something more kind and gentle? Either answer is OK, and you get to decide which option connects most with your body kindness goals.

TAKE ACTION: You close your eyes and say to yourself, "I love you. I love you. I love you," until the tightness in your chest relaxes a bit and your reaction to the photograph seems like a distant memory. Resolve to do this any time you catch yourself being mean to your body.

When it comes to body confidence, never underestimate the subconscious power of a good pep talk. Any time you catch yourself alone in the bathroom, look yourself straight in the mirror and say any (or all) of the following: "Hello, bombshell, you're doing great. I love you. It's pretty sweet when you actually stop freaking out about stuff that doesn't matter."

Once I was getting coffee with a friend when she said to me, "I don't know how you let that photo of you jumping into the pool wearing your bikini on Facebook!" Resisting the urge to spill my extra hot macchiato in her general direction, I said, "Excuse me, what?" She responded, "I'm serious. *How* do you do it? Tell me. I can't stand pictures of myself, especially in bathing suits." My response was simple and straightforward. "I don't want to delete all the memories out of my life because I don't look a certain way. Yes, there are photos of me I don't like. But I choose to be disappointed by the photo, not the person."

Tell yourself, "I am enough." And then take it a step further and say, "I am more. More than a body. More than beauty. More than how many calories I eat or what kind of exercise I do. I'm more than my boobs and butt. I'm more than an object. I'm more than what I ate for breakfast. I'm more than a pretty picture I posted on social media. I am a caring, loving, daring, powerful person. I am smart. I am worthy. I am more, and I refuse to be corseted into less."

Healing body image is a lifelong commitment. The body kindness practice supports a healthier body image, but no amount of space I can offer in this book can replace the value of support from the right helping professional, and support from people you trust. No matter how hopeless you may feel in this very moment, ask yourself if poor body image is worth the consequence of not pursuing your goals to achieve a better life.

UNSTICK YOURSELF FROM PROGRESS TRAPS

If there's one guarantee I can make to you, it's this: You will get stuck. Nobody does behavior change perfectly. Everyone messes up in ways big and small. In fact, the most successful people in the world fail repeatedly and credit their mistakes as part of what makes them great. When clients come in forlorn over a failure, I'm there to catch them with a smile and a "Hooray! I love mistakes!" Seriously. In order to make a mistake, you have to take an action first—and there is no behavior change without action. Mistakes are teachers. They help you learn and grow. I've never been more in touch with my desires, my values, and myself than when I'm making mistakes. I get worried when I'm not screwing things up. Love your mistakes. Love your failures. Every single one of them.

Based on feedback from my clients, here are the top mistakes people tend to make that prompt them to get stuck and stay there, along with what they did to unstick themselves.

Discomfort—When you get hung up on your negative thoughts and feelings, you experience emotional discomfort. To avoid that feeling, you stay in the same place, changing nothing. The fact

is, you need to experience some discomfort in order to reach your goals. The rewards far outweigh the challenges. Continue working on observing your thoughts and feelings by brushing up on mindfulness. Allow any thought or feeling to come up, and practice what you would do if you weren't uncomfortable. You will build up a familiarity and tolerance to discomfort when it arises.

Extremes—When you set unrealistic goals and expectations, you fail at something that would likely never work for you. Scale it back. Do a tiny little thing right now that's in line with your values. Spiral up and repeat it. If you're not doing what you set out to do, make it smaller. You will get there one successful action at a time.

Neglecting Values—When you don't check in to ask, "Am I living my values in this moment?" you're unaware of any disconnect and you may keep doing what you've always done, making choices that don't align with your values. You see it as lack of motivation, willpower, or ability and may give up far too soon. Reminding yourself of your values takes effort in and of itself.

You beat fears by facing them, letting them show their presence rather than trying to chase them away. In psychology they call it *exposure therapy*, in which you have planned experiences with the fearful event or feelings, until you become more comfortable with it. You feel your fear while you do the very thing that scares you. One example is my client Barb, whose numerous fears were so powerful she avoided exercise. Her father had died of a heart attack, and every time her heartbeat escalated or became irregular, she would stop immediately. She also feared being made fun of for her difficulty walking up hills, needing to take breaks, and even her appearance in workout clothes. Barb was never going to exercise regularly by avoiding it. She had to face her fears incrementally. She started by wearing a pedometer and walking more frequently in her regular clothes during her daily activities and acknowledging any movement as beneficial physical activity. She scheduled exercise in her home—dancing and cleaning, mindfully noticing that when her heart rate increased she was OK. During our sessions, we walked hills together. At all times, she was in control. I could be there to support her thoughts and feelings and suggest rests, even if she didn't request them.

Exposure to fear in a safe, controlled environment is the most effective way to move past it. **Pushing past the fear teaches your brain that most of what we fear doesn't ever happen, and even when it does—we can handle it.** The more often you repeat this process, the more effective it becomes.

Gratitude

"Happiness is the consequence of personal effort." This quote is often attributed to author Elizabeth Gilbert of *Eat, Pray, Love* and *Big Magic* fame, who has enthusiastically cultivated gratitude for years through a ten-second daily practice she calls her "Happiness Jar." Using any scrap of paper she can find, Gilbert records the happiest moment of her day and saves it. In 2013, as a way to renew her nightly ritual after a whirlwind year, she shared an image of her scrap-filled apothecary jar on social media and inspired thousands of readers to expand and adapt her idea. Gilbert calls it the simplest, least-demanding spiritual practice in her life, and her readers confirm that the results are nothing short of transformative—helping them to find the moments of happiness buried in everyday life and even forgiving themselves when they miss a day or two (or thirty)!

There are many ways you can incorporate this into your own life—from a keepsake jar or a daily note in your bedside journal to a simple dinner table conversation when each person shares the best part of their day. Gilbert's happiness project inspired me to cultivate a "Year of Kindness" practice in my own life and, not surprisingly, gratitude and happiness have grown alongside it, as I dedicate a few seconds each day to cap-turing the kindness I have given and received. I've shared these little pieces of love on social media, and I get an extra burst of warmth when people tell me my own self-gratitude helped them get through a bad moment. What I've learned most from cultivating kindness is that **acts of big kindness and small kindness toward others can make you feel the same rewarding energy for yourself.**

Gilbert adds, "I keep up this practice not as protection against dark times or denial of dark times (we cannot protect against dark times or deny their exis-tence; dark times happen, and will keep on happening) but as an act of stubborn gladness and gratitude for the strangely unfolding miracle that is my life." How often are you practicing gratitude? Can you turn it into a ritual? Ask yourself, "What's the bright side of my life despite this difficulty?" Get a few close friends to join you on a daily gratitude email. Even if you don't all contribute every day, you'll notice how one person's self-reflection on the gifts in their life makes you want to be nicer to yourself.

The Power of Intention and Affirmation

You're not going to change your habits through affirmations alone, but they can be a valuable part of befriend-ing yourself. When I was doing my self-discovery work to overcome emo-tional eating, much of my healing came through my yoga practice, where my teachers encouraged me to hold myself with love, kindness, and compassion. During that time, as I got more curious about the triggers for my emotional eat-ing, I found that the words *live with ease* came to mind frequently and brought me a sense of comfort and peace.

At the end of each yoga class, I'd meditate on my mantra. Practicing the mantra allowed me to engage with it when I needed it the most. My emotional triggers were strongest when I felt I was in a situation I wouldn't be able to han-dle. By practicing this ahead of time, my body and mind began to connect those words with the feeling of deep relaxation I felt after yoga. Each time I visualized a sort of helpless danger and used my *live with ease* mantra, it strengthened my ability to face stressful situations. I could use *live with ease* as a way of telling myself I was OK, and I would be OK. It didn't happen overnight, but I am proud to say that I beat years of emotional overeating struggles through practicing mindful body kindness and daily affirmation.

All You Need Is Love

The core body kindness pillar is love. And when all else fails, you always have the power to bring yourself back to this foundation. Love is the birthplace of forgiveness, acceptance, and compassion. When you approach change from a place of love, you become your own best friend and give yourself the same support you would offer another person who is struggling with change. This means intentionally cultivating a love for yourself, just as you are, instead of giving all your attention to the person you want to become.

BODY KINDNESS REFLECTION: Open up your journal and spend fifteen minutes thinking about self-acceptance. In what ways do you feel you are already aligned with body kindness and in what ways are you not?

"The curious paradox is that when I accept myself just as I am, then I can change."

—Carl Rogers

Part Four

Where You Belong

Deepen Your Connections

Chapter 11

Nurture Your Closest Connections

Spiral Up with Those
Who Matter Most

Philosophy

Having strong, healthy relationships is one of the best-kept secrets to achieving a happy, healthy, and meaningful life. Before we are even born, we are connecting. The sounds of life outside the womb and skin-to-skin contact shortly after birth help encourage strong emotional bonds with our parents. As we grow, we are constantly seeking out attachment and connection. Those who matter most to us can strongly influence our body kindness practice. Like many animals, we are naturally designed to "tend and befriend" one another as a caregiving way to respond to stress. Honoring your tightest connections is an integral part of transforming your habits and creating a better life.

BODY KINDNESS PILLARS
Tend and Befriend

LOVE: Growing the love you share with others can help fuel your body kindness efforts.

CONNECT: Nurturing your closest relationships can help you honor your relationship with yourself.

CARE: The care you provide to those who matter most reflects the strengths you have to take care of yourself.

You've Got a Friend

Up to this point *you* have been at the center of the body kindness philosophy—which is exactly where you should be! But what if the strength of your body kindness practice hinged on the quality of your relationships? We often view taking care of ourselves and taking care of others as mutually exclusive. Sometimes it feels like we can do only one or the other, and that if we are ambitious enough to try for both, we risk doing neither very well. "I can't take care of myself because my family needs me." Or "I need to be healthier before I can really show up and give value to this relationship." But it doesn't have to be that way.

When you spend less time in your head worrying about not being good enough, your inner voice becomes kinder and gentler, and you have more mental energy to engage with those who mean the most to you. Investing in your relationships spirals you up in energy and motivation to care for yourself. Likewise, when you make progress with body kindness, you are in the best possible place to give exactly what your relationships need—your true self: honest, real, and imperfect.

All the time and energy we put into our "health" for the sake of appearances would be better spent focusing on developing and maintaining strong relationships. Researchers say that a lack of social connections harms well-being more than obesity, high blood pressure, and smoking. Think about that. When was the last time a burger and fries with your bestie was something you did to be healthy? Go ahead, revel in a special bond as a matter of well-being!

Spiral Up

Think about one of the happiest days of your life. Who was with you? How did their presence make the moment? Whom did you share this joyful experience with after it happened? Now think about a difficult time in your life when you needed someone. How did they help you get through it? How do your closest connections strengthen your well-being, support body kindness, and help you create a better life for yourself?

Behavior change is a social process. By involving those you care about in your body kindness goals and grasping how your relationships impact your choices, you can actually strengthen your connections to others and improve your health.

Here are just a few ways your relationships can help body kindness flourish:

You make decisions about what you want to do. Friends can help with ideas and "what worked for me" recommendations when you ask.

Loved ones can give you time, permission, or other resources that help you follow through on your commitments.

They may do it with you! Behavior change is contagious. You're more likely to inspire change in others not because you twisted their arm, but because they caught your "fever" for body kindness.

Encouragement, listening, and emotional support will help you along the way. Through the normal ups and downs, they can be a source of strength and power. It's motivating to know others are behind us.

Keep friends and family in your thoughts for your own motivation to keep going. We like the idea of making others proud and serving as a role model. Do it for them (and yourself) as an expression of dedication.

The people you spend the most time with are perfect candidates for growing and spiraling up together. Seeing you happy and taking care of yourself can unexpectedly rub off on those you love. Whether it's going on a hike together or visiting the farmers' market—all the changes in your life will give you plenty to talk about. I encourage you to share your goals with friends and family, and let them know how they can support you.

Who Is on Your Post-it?

Bréné Brown says that you should be able to write the names of the people who matter the most to you on a single, small piece of paper that can fit in your wallet. This is a short list, so I hope that everyone who earns a space on yours genuinely deserves it. None of us live in an abyss, so taking the time to recognize how we are influenced by other people is essential to making body kindness a way of life. This helps in two ways. First, it encourages you to be fully present for one of the most important aspects of life—the people you love. And by paying mindful attention to these relationships, you can intentionally surround yourself with positive connections and focus on people who support your goals. These are the people who are most deserving of your time and attention. Give them your kindness freely and accept theirs in return. When an act of kindness is carried out, our brain associates it with pleasure, connection, and

Spiral Up

THE PEOPLE ON YOUR POST-IT NOTE

Fill a Post-it note with the names of those people you care about most in life, place it in your body kindness journal, and shower each person on that list with kindness. If you live with them, be intentional about unplugging from your phone when they get home and giving them the gift of your full attention. Send a *real* card in the mail, call them to just say "hello" and hear their voice, buy them a small, meaningful gift, send flowers, make special plans you can look forward to, or invite them to take a walk, just the two of you. These efforts should feel invigorating. They are not just another to-do to prove your love. Say "thank you" and mean it. Do it in your own way and on your schedule. Then take time to enjoy the upward spiral of meaningful connection.

trust. The bonus is that endorphins are released in both people involved.

Finding practical ways to cultivate mindfulness, gratitude, forgiveness, and kindness increases our sense of well-being and strengthens our connections with the people who matter most in our lives. Random acts of kindness don't have to be expensive or time-consuming, but they are always worth the effort, especially because the real reward is the happiness you and the recipient both feel. Imagine how good it feels to receive (and give) a little "just because" surprise. Reach out and touch someone's heart. Reconnect with someone who has been in your thoughts recently.

Kindness Brings People Together!

I'll be honest, I can count on one hand the number of times I have sent or received flowers. That's how I know I wasn't alone in thinking that they were frivolous and unnecessary, but that is exactly why you should send them! Recently I was taken by surprise when one of my interns sent me some thank-you flowers. Not only did they look and smell absolutely amazing, they instantly brightened up my mood. I placed my beautiful bouquet in one of the busiest rooms of the house, smiling every time I walked past them. For the next week, I got to enjoy this thoughtful gift and share it with my family. "Loren sent you those?" my husband said. "How nice of her! They look great." My three-year-old daughter enjoyed smelling them with full-lung-capacity inhales like Olaf's when he finally experiences summer flowers in *Frozen*. My two-year-old and I practiced naming all the colors at least a dozen times.

Amazed by how something that seemed so effortless could spark such great emotion, I was inspired to bring this joy to someone else. As the sender of flowers, I got pleasure out of choosing the best gift, writing the message on the card, and anticipating her reaction. But I was not prepared for the news that the floral love continued to grow. The email subject said, "You Inspired Me!" After expressing heartfelt gratitude toward me, my friend said that she sent a bouquet, too. She was feeling guilty about not spending time with someone important and she thought sending flowers was better than nothing. Lifted by the good mood my gift gave her, she took an immediate step to reconnect. Later, her friend telephoned. "You have no idea how much I needed these today. I've been so blue. Thank you for cheering me up." Getting this update from my friend made me even happier! I felt connected to a total stranger and satisfied that my kindness had played a small role in improving someone else's day. I think we were all a little high on joy for a while. While I can't prove all this flower-giving was directly responsible for anyone sticking to their body kindness goals, I'm confident the positive energy and shared upward spirals helped us all remember what matters most. That's good enough for me.

The Biology of Belonging

What many of us learned in our Psych 101 classes about Abraham Maslow's hierarchy of basic human needs still holds true: Once our basic biological needs are met (food, water, sleep, sex), the next areas we seek to fulfill are psychological needs, safety and belonging. These are all considered "deficiency needs," which means that if any of them go unmet, our health suffers. In other words, before we can hope to reach any level of long-term health, we have to pay attention to our sense of belonging and our relationships. Ignoring these important needs can lead to downward spirals of emotional health, including depression, loneliness, and isolation. And often on the way down people engage in numbing behaviors in an attempt to avoid these types of pain.

When life knocks you down, one of the most important ways you can help yourself is to rely on the strength of others. When we keep our hearts and minds open to other people, our stress levels decrease, our cardiovascular system operates more efficiently, and our vagal tone (a measurable sign of well-being) improves. The vagus nerve runs from our head to our intestines and regulates breathing, heart rate, digestion, muscle movement, and emotions. As you know, all of these body systems tend to get involved (and act up) when we feel stressed. People with a higher vagal tone are more resilient and have more mind-body strength. They are less likely to suffer from diabetes, depression, and irritable bowel syndrome, among other ailments.

The mindset "I need people and people need me" represents the powerful role our social bonds play in our health and happiness. Yet all too often we tend to isolate ourselves, saying, "I don't want to bother anyone. I'm being stupid. Nobody cares about my problems." We also get stuck in the unhealthy mindset that we *should* be able to manage alone. For a million different reasons, when we need people the most, we have trouble asking for help. Reality check: How mad would you be at your friend if she was suffering alone in silence instead of letting you in? Why is it OK for you to help others, but they can't help you? Underneath this double standard are doubts about your worthiness and what receiving help says about your character. But talking to someone you trust is one of the most effective ways of coping. Whether it's a supportive friend or a helping professional, these conversations can help prevent emotional overeating, alcohol abuse, and other self-destructive behaviors. Reaching out to others can help you sleep better at night, feeling more rested than if you were up worrying into the wee hours.

Allowing people who care about you to help is a gift you can give to them. I know that I feel honored when other people trust me enough to be a part of their support system. When someone recognizes your vulnerability and offers support, their brain is flying high on the hormone oxytocin, which tells them to find opportunities to help. It's a natural caregiving instinct we all have. You get the physical and emotional benefits of support, and people feel good about being there for you. Going through stressful experiences together makes both of your lives more meaningful, even though the experience may not be positive. Use your social support. You are never alone with your troubles unless you choose to be.

Think of at least one person you think would be willing to listen and support you the next time you are feeling overwhelmed with life. If you can think of two or three, even better! What are the qualities you see that make them a good support person? If you feel comfortable, mention to your friend or family member that you've spent some time thinking about who is supportive in your life and they are on your list. You may think this kind of support is unspoken, such as with a spouse or a best friend. But just saying out loud how you feel about asking for help will open lines of communication and strengthen your bond with this person. It's also a permission slip to engage their help when you need it.

Building Body Kindness at Home

Body kindness is not just about working on your life, it's about being in your life. Spiral up naturally by being fully engaged with your most important people. It starts with putting your phone and computer away. I'm talking to myself as much as anyone else. When I realized my husband and

Spiral Up
LOSE YOUR PHONE

. . . .

Challenge yourself to spend a weekend day without your phone. Do everything you usually do, but without your face stuck to a screen. Notice what you see. Most likely lots of people on their phones, not talking to the nail technician, checkout clerk, or their own kids out for a bite to eat. If you meet up with friends, observe what they do with their phone in your presence. Take mental notes and then later spend some time reflecting on how you felt when you saw people ignoring one another.

I were both on Facebook commenting on the same status update while sitting next to each other in silence I thought, "This is not OK." Social media may be about real life, but it's not real life. It's a life we live online. It's easily contrived to look better than reality. There's even a new buzzword called *phubbing*—a mash up of *phone* and *snubbing*. It's the act of paying more attention to your phone than the person whose company you are in. We are losing intimate connections through our overdependence on technology. **True intimacy comes from talking without distractions, making eye contact, and hugging one another— the kinds of actions that build trust, a bond for building love.** I adore social media. But at some point, you may need to power down if you're going to spiral up in your relationships.

By now, I hope you are making changes and having conversations about what you need for "me time" with your people. If you're still feeling time-trapped, you are going to need to resolve it if you want to feel free enough to take committed action toward your goals. Remember, the people closest to you stand to benefit in a big way from your changes, and as far as body kindness goes—what's good for you is good for them, too. Get with your partner and discuss the logistics of making "we time" and "me time." I find people feel so much less guilt about working on themselves when they accept that their changes help the people they care about, and when there's adequate family bonding time on the calendar, too. If you don't believe it, track it for a week. You'll see reading books, watching a movie together, family meals, and leisure activities add up. Perhaps you need to be more mindful when it's happening and savor the moment. Notice when "we time" elevates your mood, and trust that it carries over to your body kindness practice. Perhaps you need exciting surprises on your family time schedule to create some shared upward spirals and deepen your connections.

You might be pleasantly surprised at some of the supportive responses you get from your people as you begin to make body kindness a way of life. Showing special people that you value your well-being and that you believe it's never too late to change your mindset and your habits are the greatest gifts you can give them. Clients will often say to me, "Please help me be a good role model." I can't think of a better way to do that than with body kindness. Don't wait to be "ready" or in your ideal place to consider yourself a good role model—you already are. By sharing your efforts, showing your commitment to your well-being, and celebrating your strengths, you are encouraging others to do the same.

Bonding over Food

The mere act of cooking and eating together is an expression of love, and sharing food with other people can be a source of great happiness and satisfaction. Whether you're sitting down to a harried family dinner or lingering at the hot new restaurant with a group of friends, great food, and fine wine, **you create upward spirals of emotion when you spend time connecting with people over food.** It's one of the best things you can do for your mind and body.

Family mealtime has been linked to everything from lower rates of substance abuse and depression to reduced risk of developing an eating disorder and increased resiliency. Children who regularly eat meals with their family also boast higher GPAs and self-esteem, and a more robust vocabulary from all that dinnertime conversation. To be fair, it's not likely that magical roasted vegetables create this impact, but rather that families who make time for meals together are prioritizing and investing in their family relationships overall. When kids are asked whom they would like to have a meal with if they could eat with anyone, they choose their family. Not professional athletes, not celebrities, just their boring parents. This bonding and connection doesn't have to wait until the food is placed on the table. Preparing the meal also presents lots of opportunities to interact—whether it's choosing the menu, chopping the vegetables, or just chatting casually in the kitchen while one of you cooks.

Research shows that five meals together each week offer the greatest benefit, but every bit counts! The most important ingredient is time. At least one parent with one child committed to the mealtime. Can't do dinners? Try breakfast or lunchtime instead. I have one friend who meets her husband for lunch every Thursday so they can catch up and connect on a regular basis. If your schedule seems too full for meal plans, keep it simple and quick. There are more healthful prepared food options than ever before, and remember that the most important thing is the opportunity to reconnect over a meal. Everything else is details.

Even the most time-starved families can successfully make meals happen. Whatever that looks like to you, take it as a "win" and don't worry about imperfections. Maya Angelou said, "People will never forget how you made them feel"—use that as a reminder to skip any unnecessary fuss around mealtimes and focus on making others feel loved at the dinner table. This does not have to be perfect by any stretch of the imagination. Any effort to make it more meaningful boosts happiness.

Sometimes the missing "spice" in food is excitement. Your taste buds can easily get bored with "the usual," yet you lack the motivation to discover new tastes. **Since food and friends go together like peanut butter and jelly, use the excuse of social time to practice your kitchen skills.** The best kind of learning involves adventure, food, and friends. Here are three ideas that will help you create "Friendsgiving" more than once a year.

TRY A COOKBOOK CLUB

A cookbook club is a great way to enjoy all the benefits of entertaining with a fraction of the work. Instead of cooking a multicourse meal by yourself, everyone contributes. This helps enhance the communal vibe, sparks conversation, and provides the opportunity to try new dishes.

Grab a group of your favorite people—family, friends, friends that feel like family—and agree on a cookbook, type of cuisine, or some other exciting theme.

Everyone chooses a different recipe to prepare. Consider going a little beyond your comfort zone here to expand your cooking skills and get the rush of trying something new.

Bring the prepared dish and copies of the recipe to share with your crew. Enjoy trying all the food, as well as the company of your friends.

Chat about likes, dislikes, and variations. Get into a spirited competition and vote for the best dish. Winner gets a bottle of wine!

Everyone leaves with ideas for meals to add to their repertoire. (And hopefully leftovers, to start the week stocked up.)

Another easy angle, especially if you already have a book club, is to devote a session or two to food books in general, bringing food that's tied to the story or region in some way.

COOKING COMPETITION

There's a reason people love to watch cooking shows. Something always goes wrong, and those chefs are so darn creative! Why not try re-creating that "hot" kitchen environment with your family and friends? Let one person choose the ingredients and the other(s) find creative and delicious ways to use them. Choose more adventurous ingredients for more daring cooks and eaters.

A little cooking "challenge" is a great way to get your kids interested in food at age-appropriate levels. They can pick the secret ingredient for you to cook, help you come up with a recipe idea, or cook it for you all by themselves. My daughter picked sardines off the shelf. I was not going to say no to fish, but I was not happy with my challenge. Turns out those suckers blend into nothing in the food processor and add tons of flavor to pasta primavera. I'm always more inclined to put forth extra effort if it helps my kids learn without involving a computer screen. But in the end, it's good fun for everyone and it helps us all eat better.

COOKING SCHOOL

Try an in-home cooking class. My friend Karman hired a personal chef to come show a group of friends how to cook a whole delicious menu: "The chef had a seasonal menu set up—we made a green soup from spinach, watercress, and other greens, filet mignon done very simply, sweet potatoes with a lime dressing, and a blueberry and lemon tart. We cooked and baked and the chef served us outside at a beautiful table. It was probably up there on my top ten favorite meals of all time. It was so simple and good! We relaxed, learned some new things, and enjoyed cheerful conversation."

One client I work with shares "Thursday Supper" with a group of other families. They rotate houses and everyone brings a side, with the host providing the main dish. The only rule: no fancy recipes! This type of weekly community meal is a growing movement in America, where too often we are separated from our neighbors by computer screens and busy schedules.

The dinner table can act as a unifier, a place of community. Sharing a meal is an excuse to catch up and talk, one of the few times where people are happy to put aside their work and take time out of their day. And you don't have to have a family to enjoy family meals. You could create a weekly meal tradition by inviting a few friends over and asking them to each bring a friend you don't already know or haven't seen in a while.

Fitness with Good Friends

Let fitness be a relationship builder. Have a stressed-out friend you wish

MEMORABLE MEALS

SAVOR THE MOMENTS WITH THOSE WHO MATTER THE MOST

Make the most out of the daily ritual of sitting down to eat with friends, family, even coworkers.

Conversation Starters

What was the best part of your day? Who did something nice for you? What was it? What surprised you today? Good or bad? What was going on in your life a year ago today? Five years ago?

KEEP TRYING! Reluctant conversationalists will improve with time and patience. Once you start incorporating these questions into your mealtime conversations on a regular basis, everyone will find themselves thinking of how to answer as they go about their day.

SIMPLE WAYS TO SPIRAL UP

MUSIC

Take turns choosing music for mealtimes. Select tunes that set a mood without distracting from the conversation and enjoyment of the food. Bluegrass for BBQ, jazz for romance, soul music for soul food, etc.

ATTIRE

Change out of your sweats and apron. Put on a cozy sweater for comfort food or wear Grandma's pearls when you are cooking her best Italian dish.

TABLE DECOR & PLACE SETTINGS

Flowers are classic. A few pretty autumn leaves, a branch, or a tower of pinecones can be a nice surprise. Filling a pretty glass jar with acorns is a fun project for kids. Place cards with a little sketch on them make a diner feel special. Place mats and cloth napkins add color and elegance—so do the good dishes!

LIGHTING

Dimmers, candles, soft lights. Ambiance promotes calm conversation and intimacy.

you could help through a difficult time? Invite her to a yoga class. Try something new together, like indoor rock climbing or hiking out in nature (which is not only good for you, your lungs, and your mood, but it's also a very cool way for kids to learn science). Go canoeing or biking. Who cares if it's leisurely. At least you aren't on your butt carving out indentations on the sofa! Or just be playful with your younger kids. Play hopscotch in the driveway. Play freeze dance with their favorite songs—try hip-hop, salsa, and country and western stations. Put in a workout DVD and let them try it along with you. Little kids will think it's silly fun. We are all kids at heart, and our bonding time can be playful and active. If you have older kids in a sport, walk the track and get lost in music or a great book, then catch up on life during the car ride. Say yes to the opportunity to move with the people who matter.

Think of these shared experiences as one of the ways you take care of yourself or as an expression of gratitude that you can extend to other people. It could be any form of self-care you value when the opportunity arises. One of the key factors in successful bonds is the presence of rituals. The human mind and spirit thrive on consistency and familiarity—so whether you commit to weekly dinners, monthly meetings, or Sunday church—just keep showing up. Chances are, life will surprise you with what it has in store.

Time is a precious commodity, and it can often feel that the needs of others leave us no time for taking care of ourselves. We think it's just easier to let go of our needs or that it's impossible to do it all. Until you've felt the true ongoing benefits of upward spirals in your life, **it's hard to believe that taking an hour out of your day to exercise or play will help you keep up with other, more urgent things.** This can be particularly difficult if someone in the family has special needs. But if you don't take any other piece of advice from me, please trust me on this one. You have to put on your own life jacket first, even—especially—if it feels like you're all sinking.

Kristen's daughter was diagnosed with type 1 diabetes at the age of three—and if you know anything about this illness, you'll understand that her family's life changed overnight. Her daughter's life depended on constant monitoring and attention to her blood sugar. This meant lots of sleepless nights and stress for Kristen, and initially her instinct was to drop everything in her own life to keep her daughter safe. But at some point, Kristen realized that she had to prioritize her own self-care to be the mom she wanted to be. Her advice to other people in a similar situation is to remember, "It's OK to focus on yourself and give yourself time. No one is going to walk up to you and say, 'Hey, go take a break; let me help you.' You have to ask for it, and that's not a sign of weakness.

It's a sign of strength and self-worth. This is important, so I can do the amazing work I need to do. If I don't take care of myself, everything will fall apart."

The gift of practicing body kindness is that you don't have to choose between your role as a parent, spouse, employee, daughter, or friend and your own well-being. You get to do both! If you're married with kids, make a commitment with your partner to protect each other's "me time" as a united front, and don't forget the benefits of "we time"

either. Even if it's just sharing a cup of coffee before the rest of the house wakes up or a glass of wine and conversation at the end of a long week, developing rituals and habits that foster connection will strengthen your relationship and spiral up in ways you can't yet imagine. Believe me, I know it feels impossible sometimes; I'm right there with you. But taking the time to nurture that connection in advance quickly pays off in fights avoided and body kindness goals shared and achieved.

Getting Sexy On

Touching someone you care about—a hug, a caress, a kiss—creates chemical reactions in both of you, reinforced by emotions meeting a physiological need. **If just simple touching can do all this, just imagine what sex can do!** Clients don't usually expect to cover this topic when they come in to a dietitian's office, but if you really want to transform your life and use upward spirals to make it happen, then sex should be a part of the discussion. Intimacy is a basic human need that is deeply connected to happiness and well-being, and let's face it, orgasms are the ultimate upward spiral. Whether it's with a partner or on your own, this is one area of life that you can transform almost instantly without

spending a dime. If you're one of thousands of women who think they don't need sex to be happy, then please just humor me for a few pages and see how your libido responds.

Let's start with the science, because that seems to be a topic most of us are comfortable talking about. Some of the areas that we have outlined as important to body kindness include managing stress, improving sleep, and strengthening healthy relationships. Sex supports all of these. It boosts your mood and your immune system and also has the power to improve your self-esteem and body image. Not feeling sexy? My challenge to you is to do it anyway, at least once a week. There are a couple of reasons I support the "just do it" mentality when it comes to intimacy. Like any other form of exercise, sexual activity produces natural endorphins that will boost your mood and increase your likelihood of practicing self-care (even without orgasm). In addition, couples who have sex weekly report fewer arguments and higher levels of relationship satisfaction. While these studies haven't proven cause and effect (Do happy couples have more sex? Or does regular sex make couples happier?), my semi-professional opinion is that your partner is less likely to get worked up over a dent in the car when he's getting some action on a regular basis. And if you're single, this same advice applies—you will be less likely to get worked up over life when you're getting "satisfied" on the regular. Becoming aware of when your need for intimacy is being met (or not) is an important part of your physical and emotional well-being.

"I'm willing to try feathers," I said to my husband. We weren't in the bedroom yet. We were at a sex workshop at Secret Pleasures Boutique in Washington, DC. With an infant and toddler at home, our sex life was experiencing a bit of a dry spell. Maybe being tired made me less into it. Or maybe it was the six-month-old attached to my boob or hip 24/7. All I knew was I loved my husband, but I didn't feel like having sex with him and it bothered me. So here we were matching our answers from a checklist of the "dirty deeds" we'd be willing to try. The purpose was to add some sexual spice before the

clothes came off—actually talk, respect each other, and maybe surprise each other—you're into *dulce de leche* in the bedroom, too? *Check.* I learned a lot that night. First, I learned that it's unrealistic to expect that sex in real life is just like the movies. You don't have to look or feel like a *goddess* to enjoy good sex. Also, sex can be decidedly *unsexy*. Sometimes people fart, queef, and throw their backs out. Sex is silly, awkward, quiet, noisy, boring, and exciting. When you're a parent to toddlers, sex can be pretty stressful—"How can we sneak off? What if the kids hear us? Do I even have the energy for sex?" How are you supposed to get in the mood when you have to plan every second of your freedom? And even if you get started there's a good chance you're not finishing because somebody (not your partner) needs attention. As my husband says, "Nothing kills a boner like your kid knocking on the bedroom door inquiring, 'What are you doing in there?'" I also learned that sex is not "the relationship." Good relationships can endure a dry spell (thankfully!). For me, it came down to the realization that sex is not just another item on my to-do list. Sex is about connecting in the most intimate way—and feeling really f-ing good. My advice for anyone in a sex slump is simple—talk to each other. Be honest and open-minded. Just keep showing up. They make plenty of toys, games, and lubricants for everything else. And *Dora the Explorer* is a totally acceptable babysitter for a good quickie.

Spiral Up
BRINGING SEXY BACK

. . . .

Need a dose of bedroom or intimacy inspiration? Experiment with some of the following activities, and also be mindful of how mental chatter or inner dialogue affects your libido. Mindfulness can quiet your mind and help you stay focused on the physical experience of touching and being touched.

. . . .

Close your eyes and describe in your mind everything that is happening while you are interacting with your partner. If a thought bully interrupts you, kindly respond with a gentle "Thanks for the reminder; I'm busy now" and return your focus to the feeling of being touched. It may also help to focus on taking deep breaths, which will clear your mind, relax your muscles, and increase pleasure.

. . . .

Experiment with massage oils and lotions that you already have on hand, and use scented candles to add some aromatherapy to your intimate moments. Essential oils such as ylang-ylang, rose, and jasmine have aphrodisiac properties to spice up a hot bath and create an arousing, bubbly "pregame" soak.

. . . .

Sit down with your partner outside the bedroom and brainstorm a list of every possible sexual activity or adventure you can think of. Nothing is off limits. Then combine lists or trade and each person marks *yes*, *no*, or *maybe* next to each item on the list. You can search for a premade list online for extra ideas. Or do what I did and let a qualified sex-ed teacher lead the way.

. . . .

Call a temporary truce with your body. Even if you're not quite ready to lovingly embrace every curve, jiggle, and wiggle on your glorious body, make a commitment to smile more during sex and act like someone who thinks she is fabulous. We've all faked an orgasm once or twice to boost his ego; now it's time to do yourself the same favor. Focus on the fun. Feel the love, and when all else fails—fake it 'til you make it. You don't have to love every square inch of your body to get pleasure out of it.

Lovers' Dinner Menu

Swap your whip for a whisk, throw on *only* a sexy ruffled apron, and let the seducing begin! A steamy cooking session with your lover combines the two most pleasurable things in life: food and love.

Try this sexylicious menu full of aphrodisiac foods to get your blood flowing and your heart racing.

FOREPLAY COURSE

BLUEBERRIES AND DARK CHOCOLATE Blueberry skins have resveratrol, a powerful antioxidant that can increase blood flow, and dark chocolate has tryptophan, which becomes the neurotransmitter serotonin to induce relaxation and sexual arousal.

RAW OYSTERS Oysters—and other zinc-rich foods like shrimp—can help boost sex drive and increase sperm production. Researchers have discovered two amino acids in raw oysters that are particularly effective at boosting libido in anyone who dares to consume them.

STIMULATION COURSE

ARUGULA WITH WATERMELON AND GOAT CHEESE Arugula is loaded with magnesium and watermelon contains citrulline. Both of the compounds relax blood vessels—they work like Viagra! The aroma and taste of goat cheese makes your brain release phenylethlyamines—the hormones of love. It's like sex *before* the sex.

THE BIG O COURSE

FILET MIGNON There's something about red meat cooked perfectly that arouses many a carnivore. Protein-rich lean red meat boosts levels of dopamine and norepinephrine in men and women, increasing urges to seek more pleasurable rewards—like sex! Add a little something extra to the meal with a glaze made from balsamic vinegar, red wine, and a dash of salt and pepper.

ROASTED POTATOES WITH CHILI PEPPER Potatoes are high in potassium, which regulates your blood pressure. Chili peppers turn up the heat on your metabolism and heart rate, releasing exercise-like endorphins and causing a similar energetic, floating feeling to carry you into the bedroom.

Solo Sexy Times

Who said you need a lover to feel the love? Nothing says you enjoy being good to yourself like a little alone time in the bedroom. Self-pleasure can be a very healthy way to explore your own body, from taking the time to gently caress your skin with botanical oils to playing around with your lady parts. And it feels good! Even at very young ages, we find our vaginas, start rubbing around, and realize it's a pleasurable sensation, even if it's not sexual in nature. Yet many women think it's somehow dirty or unnecessary. I disagree. Being intimate with yourself is a form of deep connection and discovery, which are essential elements of body kindness.

If the subject of masturbation makes you uncomfortable, that's even more reason to get started. You are a grown woman, and your body is capable of bringing you amazing pleasure. It's time to really see what she can do! Try an experiment—*seven days of self-love.* Set aside five to fifteen minutes a day, for seven days straight, to explore self-pleasure. No excuses and no quitting. If you have difficulty getting started, maybe a glass of wine will help you relax on days one or two. But ideally, you will use this time to be fully present and connect with your own sexual energy. You can do this in the bedroom, the shower, or anywhere else you feel comfortable. Consider buying yourself a new "toy" or carefully repurposing that neck massager your cousin bought you for Christmas—you can even do this fully clothed. For some extra fun at the end of the week, ask your partner to watch. But no touching until your "me time" is fully complete. (Just kidding—if it leads to sex you really want, all the better!) For the record, I tried out every recommended activity and Spiral Up in this book. This literal "self-love" activity was by far my most challenging and most rewarding of them all. Turns out that just like any habit, I needed to be open-minded and consistent. The first few days it took *real* dedication. I set zero expectations—only to complete the task in the name of "book research." When the week was over, I had a whole new appreciation for my body and my skill set for stress reduction!

Communicating Effectively with People Who Matter

You are strongly influenced by your environment and the people you spend most of your time with. That's why Part One and Part Two of this book were dedicated to helping you understand what impacts your choices so you can make more meaningful ones. Like all relationships, there are ups and downs. Things don't always go the way you want or need. Think of how much interactions with others can potentially trigger that internal criticism to play nonstop in your head. "You're tuned in to *You Suck Radio*. Don't touch that dial! We're going to make you feel like crap all night long." (Cue downward spiral of emotion and self-sabotage.)

For better or worse, your connections with other people matter to you. You care about what they think. You care about the strength of your relationships. But when you practice body kindness you also care about yourself. As you work on creating a better life, people who know you best will see a different side of you. **The people in your relationships can be your strongest cheerleaders or your most powerful saboteurs.** It's worth taking time to consider how these people impact your decisions and actions, if only to be aware of potential allies or challenges on your journey.

Hopefully, the people you love most will be your greatest supporters, and some people will even be drawn to change along with you. But you may have to be patient with people while they adjust to your new way of being. Some people will want to be supportive but may not know how. Others may resent the positive changes they see in you. I've even had clients say they were afraid of being an "outsider" when they made improvements in their eating habits. Others have avoided making progress toward their

goals because they don't want to hurt anyone's feelings and they are afraid of how someone close to them may respond. It might be helpful (or necessary) to set some expectations for how your relationships could be impacted by the changes you are making. You are in charge of determining who you want to involve in your journey. What you say and how you say it can make all the difference.

Asking for Support

Do you need support, be it a pep talk or someone to work out with or someone to help hold you accountable for taking action on your goals? The way you do this is by sharing your goal, asking for help, and explicitly telling a friend what to do. **"Would you please check in with me on my goals? Ask me how I'm doing and if you can help. You don't have to be the police or anything. Just be there for me."** Please do not ask anyone to be the cops. It's not fair to put the onus of monitoring your choices and goals on someone you love. And it's unacceptable if they try to do this without being asked. There is such a thing as bad support, and it's crucial you get the kind of support you need. This calls for open, honest communication, and you may need to develop a strategy for how to handle unsolicited, unwelcome, and unhelpful advice. Sometimes just expressing gratitude and then ignoring what people say might be the best approach. Just because you thank someone for offering advice doesn't mean you have to follow it! Some of my clients have a real problem with shrugging off a hurtful comment. Besides belting out "Let It Go," I tell them to visualize scooping up the conversation in their hand and then blowing it away like they're blowing out birthday candles. Here's the reality about relationships: You can do everything in your power and sometimes it's still not enough. You could have the most clear and organized plan for setting boundaries, and it flies right over the other person's head. They just don't get it. At some point, it's counterproductive to expect that other people will always respect your boundaries and do exactly what you want. If they are going to stay in your life, you'll need to accept that you are who you are and they are who they are. You can be in two different places and still love each other. Maybe there will always be a part of your relationship that disappoints you. That's OK. You can't be willing to trade in all your values and goals to fudge the scenario you wish would be there. Even if you did, there would still be conflict and misunderstandings. Sometimes our parents, best friends, and siblings can't be what we want or need, but we have to carry on. The best you can do is stay committed to body kindness, lovingly set boundaries, and gently point out when other people are not respecting them.

Setting dialogue boundaries can be as simple as remembering your ABCs: *Answer, Bridge, Conclude*. Give them an honest answer, bridge to something you actually want to discuss, and end the conversation. Period. Full stop.

Body Talk

Appearance is deeply ingrained as a badge of "worthiness" in our culture. If someone close to you says, "You need to lose weight because I'm concerned for your health," this can be very hurtful. Remember that most people mistakenly associate weight with health. Here's your opportunity to correct it. For a person who matters, you can say "thank you" and something along the lines of "I'm proud of what I'm doing to take care of myself. I'm focusing on my habits, which is the right way to work with your genetics for better health." Give them a few examples of your changes if you would like. Or you can say, "You can't tell how healthy a person is by looking at them so please stop commenting on my body." If you want to put more energy into educating them, you can share that weight bias is not helpful in motivating behavior changes, and direct them to the Health at Every Size principles (I'll share more about that in the next chapter).

Positive Weight Loss or Appearance Comments

Their heart may be in the right place. They notice something's different about you. Maybe they notice you are happier, more confident, or energized, but what they usually say is, "You look great. Have you lost weight?" Some people practicing body kindness lose weight or their shape changes even when it's not the primary goal, and they get comments from others. In embracing the principles of body kindness, they aren't sure how to respond to weight-oriented compliments. Regarding the change in appearance, it takes a body up to a year to stabilize. It can take nearly as long for new healthful habits to become ingrained. If you're loving the appearance changes, gently remind yourself of your values, how your life has become better over time, and that appreciating your appearance is just part of your transformation (and, I'd like to think, amazing progress on self-acceptance!). When someone is genuinely trying to give you a compliment, it's always OK to say "thank you" first. But this is an amazing opportunity for you to mentor someone. Really let them know how you feel. "I'm actually not focused on a weight loss goal, and I have never felt better."

Scales of (In)Justice

I don't like to involve scales in body kindness unless there is a medical priority involving physical health. I think the ultimate in body trust is noticing changes without the numbers. When the number on the scale becomes the motivating factor, the value becomes weight loss, and that feels like dieting to me. Put trust in the process and put the scale in the closet.

"WHAT'S YOUR SECRET?" TYPE QUESTIONS

Use humor and say, "Oh, it's called being good to yourself. Seriously, it's not a diet." Then give them some examples of what you are doing.

TALKING TO A "DIET-CRAZED" FRIEND

"I'm not interested in _____. That just doesn't work for me. I'm working on healthful living without rules."

FOOD PUSHERS

You want to practice intuitive eating, but you feel a voice inside your head say, "Eat to make them happy," or perhaps they actually say, "You'll hurt my feelings if you don't eat this." This is simpler than most people think. Remember that food *is* love, and one of the ways people show kindness is through giving you food. Not to mention that maybe the version of you they are used to never says no. But now you care about tuning in to your body and you're trying really hard to set food boundaries based on your needs. It's important to you to practice this skill, but you don't want to make Grandma cry either. Give her gratitude. "Thank you! This looks wonderful. It smells great. [Insert other small talk if it fits, like 'How do you make it?', 'Is it a family recipe?', etc. Show you are interested in the offering.] You know, I'm not hungry right now, but I would love to try some later. Can you save some for me?" Most people will say "sure," or maybe the first few times you'll get a snarky comment, but then people learn that sometimes you say no to food and it's not a rejection of them. (Be sure to let your people-pleaser voice know the same.)

Stormy Relationships

Communicating effectively may involve difficult conversations and choosing forgiveness as a way of healing your own personal issues. Despite your best efforts, there will inevitably be challenges in your most valued relationships. Staying aligned requires give-and-take and acknowledgement that all relationships naturally have ups and downs. And just the way we learn to accept that struggles will come in our inner growth, the same is true for our interactions with other people. If we accept that there will be arguments and misunderstandings in life, then it's easier to be patient when they do happen, which makes the path to forgiveness and reconciliation a much shorter journey.

What if a defunct relationship is keeping you from moving toward your body kindness goals? That's a flag that something needs your attention and you may need some outside help. As humans we make mistakes, we hurt and get hurt. Forgiveness is accessible to you when you are ready. You will feel lighter as your heavy heart is lifted, freeing you up to move on.

Is there someone you need to forgive before you can move on to fully experience joy? Transgressors may not even say sorry, but you don't need them to in order to forgive. You do yourself a disservice by holding on to resentment and hard feelings. We often carry around hurt for years, thinking it does little to impact our daily lives, but internalized pain has long-term emotional and physical consequences. The path to forgiveness means you free yourself from the emotional weight of holding a grudge. And with forgiveness comes the freedom and joy to finally become the person you are meant to be. This is a gift you give to yourself, not to the person who may have done wrong.

My forty-six-year-old client Erica, who is the mother of two teenagers, struggled with low self-esteem, guilt, and poor body image for decades before coming to my office. Initially she was very reluctant to give up restrictive eating. Even though she's a physical fitness trainer, she continues to be at war with her body, and fighting through low-carb diets often led to secret binges on mac and cheese. Her inner voice was unrelenting: "You're worthless, ugly, out of control." When unpacking the root of these beliefs and talking about why she started dieting at puberty, Erica instantly identified hurt and pain from her relationship with her mom. I asked her to write a letter to her mother and bring it to the next session. Here's an excerpt:

Dear Mom,

Somewhere in the journey to lose weight, you lost yourself. You lost the importance of NOT dieting and accepting yourself. You taught me that thin = best. Somewhere along the way, your constant bad-mouthing to yourself made its way into my head, and those negative thoughts told me over and over that in order to be happy I have to be thin. I love you, Mom, but I am angry at you for that. I get angry that you seem to judge

others because of their size. I am embarrassed to eat an entire meal in front of you because you have pushed your plate aside, saying, "OH THIS IS JUST TOO MUCH FOOD!!" I am trying to move past all of this, Mom, and I will do it. But for heaven's sake, I am a grown woman and I battle with these stupid, unwarranted negative feelings about myself way too much!!! And yes, I do blame you a little. It's your job to instill in your kids the knowledge that they will always be good enough, that they should never look at themselves in the mirror and see only negative. I am determined to instill in my kids feelings of worthiness and positivity that have nothing to do with how they look. I hate to say it, Mom, but I don't want to do to them what you did to me.

Erica has been holding on to a tremendous amount of anger toward her mom and shame about herself. She felt incapable of being a good role model to her kids and mentor to her personal training clients. Erica's unresolved stormy relationship with her mom also interfered with her resolve to stop dieting once and for all. She needed to let herself leave the past behind and forgive her mom, even if just on a piece of paper her mom would never see.

Forgiveness is powerful, but it might not always be possible, and the better decision may be to choose to end the relationship, whatever that looks like to you. If you're waiting to forgive someone in order to move forward, consider the consequences of what you miss out on by waiting for an apology or wishing the problem would go away. Use the universal body kindness question, but instead of asking whether the behavior creates a better life, ask about the *relationship*. Is this relationship working to make your life richer, fuller, and more meaningful? Does it help you get the life you want for yourself? Does it help you be the person you want to be? If the answer is no, consider what needs to change. What kind of boundaries could you set with this person? Maybe they are doing the best they can, but it just doesn't meet your needs. How can you move on anyway, despite the disappointment and transgressions?

Growing is a part of life. Body kindness offers a multitude of ways you can grow together. The most important lesson is that you can't separate your self-care plan from your family-and-friends plan. Being with the ones you love, through highs and lows, is part of how you're good to yourself. As you make positive changes, you will be able to offer more—and that's why we are in relationships: to give.

- -

BODY KINDNESS REFLECTION: What actions would you like to take to strengthen your relationships? What changes may need to occur in your relationship dynamics in order to progress in body kindness? Do you need to forgive anyone in order to move on?

- -

"My humanity is bound up in yours, for we can only be human together."

—Desmond Tutu

Chapter 12

Build Your Body Kindness Tribe

Your "People" Will
Inspire You

Philosophy

A commitment to engage in fulfilling experiences with like-minded people makes practicing body kindness truly life-changing. When we transform our lives, we impact the world around us. Volunteering, helping others through difficulties, and sharing kindness create a sense of purpose in life that makes a number on the scale seem meaningless. When you have a sense of "belonging," you automatically spiral up, and it's easier to stay committed to your body kindness goals. So this chapter is dedicated to helping you identify and nourish the connections that will help you come alive. If it feels like you don't "fit" any-where, it may just be that you haven't found your tribe. Seek out people and places where you can be your true self, and when you find them, nurture those connections. Becoming more aware of our place in the world also helps keep day-to-day challenges in perspective and strength-ens our resilience.

BODY KINDNESS PILLARS
Belonging Creates a Meaningful Life

LOVE: Express love for yourself and the world through experiences that give you a sense of purpose and meaning.

CONNECT: Feeling connected to the world fills your need to belong and creates upward spirals of energy in your life.

CARE: You are naturally motivated to care for others, which helps you care for yourself.

How Helpful Is Your Tribe?

Part of the human experience is the need to feel our place in this world and to believe that we have a role in making it better. This sense of purpose is highly motivating and keeps us pursuing new experiences and growth opportunities. We take comfort in an optimistic view that life is meaningful, which energizes us to continue with our lackluster day-to-day responsibilities. Then when we have "peak experiences"—moments when we feel intense joy, wonder, awe, and ecstasy. We get inspired, strengthened, renewed, and transformed. This upward spiral pulls you into a state of being that you may have never even imagined for yourself. It chose you, not the other way around. When do you feel most connected to the world, with a sense of meaning, purpose, and vitality?

What moments give you the feeling that you're making the most out of life? It's not necessarily perfect, but where do you feel at ease?

For the benefit of using body kindness to create a better life, you need to shore up your tribe, let go of distracting connections, and free up the time and energy to create the kinds of meaningful experiences you want to have. You can put plans in place to nurture your connections and your own body kindness practice at the same time, growing together.

We all belong somewhere, but not necessarily everywhere. As you evolve, so do your needs and personal interests. As you begin to make changes based on the values and goals that are important

Spiral Up

Think of a time when being with a group of people left you feeling energized, inspired, or motivated. Maybe it was a retreat, workshop, or a memorable event that made an impact. How often do you get a chance to connect with people who help you create a better life? How does belonging to a "tribe" help you practice body kindness?

to you, the people you surround yourself with play an important role. For example, if you spend a lot of time with friends who focus exclusively on weight loss as a measurement of success, then it might be difficult for you to fully embrace body kindness. This chapter will help you identify how you are influenced by the communities you are a part of and help you make choices about what you want your tribe to look like in the future. This doesn't mean you have to kick everyone out of your life who doesn't support your body kindness goals, but you get to decide how much and in what ways to interact with people who aren't on your Post-it but remain in your life.

Human beings are creatures of comfort, convenience, and habit—this means we don't always spend much time thinking about who we spend time with. We get so accustomed to interacting in a certain way that we never stop to question if the influence of others is positive or negative. Sometimes even situations that appear to be supportive can be deceiving—like a friend who loves you, but complains all day about other people. Or a workplace that boasts flashy perks like well-stocked fridges and an in-house physician, but also expects you to be available for work 24/7. When the fit is not right, you compromise your opportunities for growth—so it's worth questioning where, how, and with whom you spend your time.

Did you know that statistically speaking, about one in four people are not going to like you no matter what you do? One of my most people-pleasing clients told me that learning to accept this changed her life. "What a relief to just stop worrying about them," she said. **She began labeling saboteurs in her life NMP ("Not My People") and she used it as a tool to quickly identify when she wasn't really in the presence of her tribe.** With this mindset, she was able to accept their differences instead of feeling inadequate. This freed up mental energy to focus on people who enhanced her well-being.

My friend Pam was once in a book club that left her counting the minutes until it was over. Everyone in the group was very nice and inclusive, but they spent more time complaining about work than talking about literature. After several meetings, she realized that while it was nice to have a monthly night out with friends, there were many people in her life who she didn't get to see often enough. So she quit the club, but kept the date marked on the calendar and started filling the time slot with different people each month. During the time she would have been at book club, she began to renew friendships and connections with other interesting people and activities. She also set a professional goal to meet, talk with, or visit at least one inspiring person each week, even just for fifteen minutes. This was a powerful way to keep her heart and mind open to a variety of influences and positive energy. It's way better than yawning at book club.

Spiral Up
WEED YOUR GARDEN TO LET IT FLOURISH

If you have ever planted flowers or vegetables, you know it's necessary to get rid of the weeds so your plants can reach their full potential. Think of your social circle and relationships as a community garden. Are there any weeds? Trust your instincts and get curious about where you are spending your time and energy. Choose healthy interactions over draining ones in order to give your spirit room to grow. Just like you did with your close connections, ask yourself the universal body kindness question: "Is my involvement helping create a better life for myself?" You might find some reasons to stay involved, but make sure it's worth it and not just a struggle to walk away. If you try to be everywhere, you're nowhere. If you say yes to this group, what will you say no to? Does that change your answer? Journal about at least one weed and the benefits of walking away. Acknowledge that it's not serving to create a better life. Maybe you take a break for a few months and re-evaluate. Or give yourself permission to flee immediately!

Finding a Non-Dieting Home

Detoxing people from diets is where I belong, and not just because of my own past experiences when I wronged myself. I'm sad for the girl I was, who tried to diet her way down to ninety-nine pounds, telling herself she could handle her hunger pangs and that not eating was a sign of strength. I wronged my clients by participating in the diet, blame, and shame game, perpetuating the oppressive culture that had created me. I needed to apologize, forgive myself, and ask for forgiveness from the people I hurt. Then something changed in one of my most valued relationships that would put me on a path of great healing and alter my life forever.

When I changed careers from nonprofit management to become a registered dietitian, it was because I genuinely wanted to help people. Based on my own history of dieting and exercise, I seriously thought the way to do that was by giving my clients meal plans, calorie counts, and exercise assignments. Long before Fitbit and Jawbone were even a twinkle in anyone's eye, I strapped Body Media monitoring devices on clients' arms like a GPS tag on a dog. Clients trusted me to track every morsel of food that passed their lips, every step they took (or didn't), and even count minutes of sleep. I thought this level of supervision was the missing motivation my clients needed to change their habits. There were some early warning signs that my approach wasn't working, but in October 2013, I got a wake-up call I will never forget.

Just two days before running my second marathon, I answered the phone to hear: "Hi, is this Rebecca Scritchfield? This is Katy from St. Rose hospital in Henderson. I'm calling about your mother." In that instant, my entire world shifted as I learned that my mom had suffered a heart attack while driving on the freeway. Thankfully she survived the crash and didn't hurt any other drivers, but she would need emergency quadruple bypass surgery. Desperate to hug my mom, I flew to Las Vegas immediately to help take care of her. When I arrived, I found out she had heart disease and diabetes. She would need medications, cardiac rehabilitation, and a complete lifestyle change. While helping her begin what would become a long recovery process, I had plenty of time to reflect. "How did we get here?"

One thing I knew for sure was that my mom's eating habits were all over the place. She openly identified as an emotional eater, as if it was something she had no control over. Sometimes she acted like it was even a good thing. I don't blame her for this mindset one bit. I wasn't exactly ringing the alarm bells that eating your emotions could be bad for your health. It was just who she was. But my mom's eating patterns were restrictive, too. Growing up, I came to learn a diet would be around the corner, perfectly timed with big life events. My mom lost and gained the same hundred pounds at least twice in her life, and her weight often fluctuated by double-digit increments. I thought back to the time she came home and proudly shared that she had been named "queen" of our local TOPS chapter for the most dramatic weight loss in the shortest time period—TOPS stood for Taking Off Pounds *Sensibly*. (Yeah, right.) She was the queen all right—the queen of dieting. I could always tell if she was on the wagon or off based on our refrigerator. When the pig magnet with "A Minute on the Lips, A Lifetime on the Hips" appeared, she was cutting calories again, sometimes barely eating anything at all.

After that terrifying phone call years ago, I was convinced my mom had dieted her way to an unhealthy state—physically and emotionally—which culminated in a heart attack and the diagnosis of both diabetes and heart disease. To be sure, I don't blame dieting for *causing* her heart attack. It's never one thing. I'm sure genetics, smoking, and stress played their parts. But the dieting was the devil that pretended to be her savior. Meanwhile, it ruined her metabolism, increased her food cravings, and disrupted her connection to her body.

Dieting was my mom's version of how to be healthy—except it wasn't. When she wasn't dieting, she didn't know how to be healthy. Layer that with the learned behavior of emotional eating and you have yourself one poisonous cocktail.

As I went through this "awakening," preparing my mom heart-healthy, diabetes-friendly meals, I declared dieting my new enemy. I became obsessed with finding out if my suspicions were correct. Was dieting really what I thought it was—a big waste of time? I was confused and angry. I almost didn't want to be right about this because this new mindset was in complete contrast with my life's work. I took people's hard-earned money under a misapprehension—a big one. Dieting does not work to make people healthier or lose weight in the long run. Yet, I was actively participating in a system that offered false hope of a better life through weight loss, not health. In the weeks following her heart attack, my mom and I poured our souls out and cried our eyes out. By the time I left to return home, I was fully committed to changing who I was. I no longer wanted to be the person who profited from perfectionism. I wanted to be the kind of person who helped empower people to learn, grow, love themselves, love their habits, to appreciate the process of changing. I was scared, lost, and uncertain about the future. How do you "teach" people not to diet? I had no idea what I was going to do. I just knew I was done strapping armbands to people and saying, "Good luck! I'll be watching."

Taking time to reflect on my values completely changed the trajectory of my personal and professional choices. When I decided to stop calorie counting and diets, I really didn't know how to do my job anymore. I had to start over. What would I do if a client wanted to lose weight? I was afraid nobody would call me anymore if I didn't promise weight loss. The transformation didn't happen overnight. I started by changing the wording on my website, reading books, attending workshops, asking my peers, trying things out on myself first, and bouncing ideas off friends and clients.

In *The Book of Forgiving*, Desmond Tutu says one way to seek forgiveness is by making a difference in the community you caused distress. You give to it, and it gives back. My work now is part of what makes my life meaningful. Every thank-you means something—like my client's husband, Mark, who wrote to me, *Thanks for giving me my wife back.* Or the mom who said, "I had the best day at the pool—in my bathing suit—*no cover-up!*" And the photos posted by the mother of full-term triplets who didn't believe she could gain the weight she needed *and* love herself. Every time I connect with someone I see myself. I'm sixteen, vulnerable, and searching for confidence. I see my mom getting knocked down by the diet culture. I see my girls—so innocent and pure—as my chance to make things right. And I see you, too. You are not alone. I have made mistakes in the past, and this is how I keep moving forward. I know I'm right where I belong. I do it for myself, my family, and anyone else who wants to be here.

Build Where You Belong

The more you embrace the body kindness manifesto, the more blatantly obvious it will be how twisted our appearance-focused, deprivation-driven culture has become. You will want your tribe, your people, your army to have your back when it's December 31 and you're *realllly* thinking about that New Year's cleanse. You need to gut-check opinions on the latest health and wellness trends. You want to read helpful information from sources you can trust.

Your body kindness tribe starts with you. Based on where you're at right now, what works for you and what doesn't? If you did not fully do the diet detox from the introduction, now is your chance. Look at the groups you identified as "weeds" earlier in this chapter (page 260). With ideas for your new tribe in mind, it will be even more clear when

GOOD VIBES WITH GOOD TRIBES

How do you know you're in the presence of a body kindness tribe member? Follow these clues:

1.
You feel like you belong, not like it's a struggle to fit in.

2.
They'll call you out on your BS—and you'll return the favor.

3.
They know what they stand for and they share their beliefs freely.

4. Tribe members are trustworthy.

5.
Your tribe members give support, encouragement, and a listening ear willingly, and you feel inspired to give it right back.

6. When it comes down to it, they make you want to be a better person.

7.
They challenge you in good ways—helping you test your own limits and realize the depth of your personal strengths.

8.
You don't have to personally know everyone in your tribe. These are clues you've spotted an influencer tribe member:

You quote them often.

You feel like their "student," like you could learn a lot from them.

You want to know who they're reading and who inspires them, to expand your influencer network.

You read their articles and social media feeds, liking, loving, and sharing their message with others.

something doesn't fit. You can "tidy up" and decide that if it doesn't help you create a better life, you'll toss it in the diet dumpster. Do it now—you'll feel so much better.

Think of the people you put on your Post-it note. Who from that list really understands you? Maybe one of them gave you a copy of this book or told you about it. Those are your people! You're already aligned. Who else shares your interests, cares about your well-being, and serves as a good filter of trends? Reach out, make plans, invite them over for a body kindness party. Cook, walk, do yoga, relax, and chat about what you're doing and how it's going. You don't need to pay to join a group so you can all get on a scale in front of one another. You just need each other!

Besides friends old and new, support the influencers and experts who share your point of view. I have a few ideas to get you started. My culinary she-roes are Ellie Krieger and Nigella Lawson. I highly recommend them for cookbooks and other help you may need in the kitchen beyond balanced plates. Ellie Krieger is a registered dietitian, mom, award-winning chef, and TV show host. She came to influence me at just the right time. I'll never forget when I heard her say, in a matter-of-fact response to a reporter's question, something along the lines of, "Sugar is just another ingredient, and it can be used to help make good-for-you foods taste even better." It seems silly now, but this was a lightbulb

moment for me. I felt so free! My plain oatmeal tasted a lot better with a touch of brown sugar. Nigella Lawson gets my stamp of approval because she has spoken out against the cringe-worthy term "clean eating," saying that "it implies that any other form of eating is dirty or shameful." Her food philosophy centers on enjoyment, not overindulging. "There are times when you need a slice of cake." (I agree, Nigella!) My fitness tribe consists of people like Jessamyn Stanley, yoga enthusiast and fat femme, whose body can take the shape of yoga poses I've been dreaming about for years, and Anna Guest-Jelley, founder and CEO of Curvy Yoga, an online inspiration and training portal for yoga students and teachers. The Body Positive Fitness Alliance is a network of trainers who are dedicated to a better fitness experience focused on full health and quality of life as opposed to extreme, potentially harmful workouts. You can search for a trainer on their website or ask around on your favorite online communities. Keep in mind that you may value an influencer and still notice she says something that doesn't jive with your beliefs, such as a weight or appearance comment that doesn't make sense or even makes you angry. Nobody is perfect. You'll have to judge overall—does having this person in your life (or email inbox) help you create the happy and healthy life you want?

Look to organizations and initiatives that care about well-being. The Health at Every Size (HAES) principles were created by a group of experts and advocates at the Association for Size Diversity and Health, which cares about fighting weight stigma. The HAES principles embrace a holistic definition of health to include size diversity, health enhancement, respectful care, eating for well-being, and life-enhancing movement. Other groups I admire and respect include The Body Positive, Beauty Redefined, Adios Barbie, and The Body Is Not An Apology. The documentaries *Miss Representation* and *The Illusionists* should be shown at every college campus, sorority, and church event to help open up eyes to the unrelenting pressures placed on women to value their appearance over anything else. Social media has become an exciting way to find your "tribe" and use your voice to advocate for things you care about. There are free Facebook groups full of potential tribe members, offering support for intuitive eating, body positivity, and the like. Many eating disorder treatment centers offer community support. You don't have to have gone through eating disorder treatment to benefit from positive messages on social media or group events that may lead to meeting more tribe members. We're all in this together—and together will be how we will all change.

Another way to spread the body kindness love is by taking care of yourself and teaching the young people in your life that what they see on magazine pages and in TV commercials is a lie. Create a definition of beauty that goes beyond physical description. Try not to insult yourself (or other women) in front of your children. Each time you look at a scar or a stretch mark, embrace the story of what created it and cherish the depth and texture that each experience has brought to your life. Before we can insist that society sees us as more than objects, we have to be willing to do that for ourselves.

If you're tired of the objectification and sexualization of women in mainstream media and marketing campaigns, I encourage you to fight back. Make a conscious effort to spend your time and money supporting companies that offer a more diverse notion of what it means to be feminine and beautiful. According to the American Psychological Association, this isn't just a matter of personal opinion, it's a life and death issue. Increased incidences of depression, eating disorders, and low self-esteem among young girls have been directly linked to early exposure to sexualized media images. Unfortunately, as a culture we are becoming more and more desensitized to ads that espouse a frighteningly young, monochromatic version of beauty and that sensationalize violence against women. And with the modern use of Photoshop, the images we see of women are further from reality than ever.

In a speech on body confidence, actress Gabourey Sidibe talked about how often she gets asked, "Gabourey, how are you so confident?"

"If I hadn't been told I was garbage, I wouldn't have learned how to show people I'm talented. And if everyone had always laughed at my jokes, I wouldn't have figured out how to be so funny. If they hadn't told me I was ugly, I never would have searched for my beauty. And if they hadn't tried to break me down, I wouldn't know that I'm unbreakable. **So when you ask me how I'm so confident, I know what you're really asking me: How could someone *like me* be confident? Go ask Rihanna, a**hole!"**

Award-winning singer Adele takes home a bunch of Grammys and all people can focus on is her size. Then she starts exercising ahead of a tour and all they can talk about is her "amazing weight loss transformation." What about her talent? One of my favorite musicians, Pink, does beautiful aerial dancing as part of her performances, but she was criticized for supposed weight gain when she was photographed at a cancer benefit. She defended herself with, "*I am perfectly fine, perfectly happy, and my healthy, voluptuous, and crazy strong body is having some much deserved time off. Love, cheesecake.*"

It's time to take back our bodies and our brains and fight against the oppression. We need to shift our own inner dialogue and seek out people, products, and activities that support a kinder, more diverse and authentic version of beauty. Let's send celebrities some love when they reject the beauty and body standards thrown at them. Support the magazine stories and blog posts that promote inclusivity of all bodies.

Vote with your dollar. Retailers are listening. In January 2016, after decades of feedback from women around the world, Mattel finally released Barbie dolls that reflect a more diverse image of beauty. I'm so excited that my daughters have more options for who belongs in the Dream House that I'm tempted to buy one of every shape, color, and size! We need more companies willing to create and advertise products that represent how bodies actually look, not how society wants them to look. We need more brands like Dove, whose pioneering 2006 video *Evolution* exposed the great lengths advertisers go to in order to get the "perfect" look using makeup, Photoshop, and other artificial means. Support the brands you believe act with compassion and represent your values.

The Power of Collaboration
in Body Kindness

Establishing a group of people with shared goals will give you a place to experience, learn, and practice body kindness. You can help one another set goals, celebrate accomplishments, and share challenges. Group support leads to more upward spirals of energy, and the willingness to be vulnerable with others is a powerful tool for growth. If you're lucky, you will find someone in the group who's not afraid to call you out or challenge you in a loving way. These kinds of relationships can serve as an external guide to help you reconnect with your inner voice.

A sense of connection and belonging can be a tremendous source of encouragement when it comes to making positive life changes. In group-based, health-focused challenges everybody wins, especially when our competitive nature gets involved. Everyone seems to do better with shared goals and peer motivation. My clients value their health groups because "It gives me accountability partners. I have something to look forward to that excites me, which is important when I'm unsure about the challenge that lies ahead. I know I'm not the only one going through this. It's more fun with someone else."

My sister Laura, who proudly sips coffee from a mug that reads "If You're Pushing Forty That's Exercise Enough," helped pull a 747 airplane down the runway at Dayton International Airport once. Several people in her office were banding together to do this outrageous activity to help raise awareness and financial support for a colleague's daughter who was newly diagnosed with type 1 diabetes. She had already been having "the talk" with herself about needing to get more exercise. When this opportunity came up it served as just the kick in the pants she needed. Everyone trained for the pull by forming teams, walking together at lunch, and logging their steps from home. My sister confessed, "There is no way in hell I would have done all the exercise I did for this challenge on my own. But now that I'm doing it, I don't want to stop. **I'm already looking for the next challenge. I'm the one asking my coworkers, 'What crazy thing can we do next?'"**

And you don't even need to leave your house to reap the benefits of group collaboration. One of my sister's most dependable workout routines is a weekly elliptical date with friends by video or phone chat. No gym membership

Spiral Up
A YEAR OF
GROUP FITNESS CHALLENGES

How would you like to take the pressure off setting personal fitness goals for a whole year? By coordinating fitness efforts with a few friends, you can share the load and keep the motivation going all year long. Start by inviting up to eleven friends, relatives, coworkers, or even friends of friends, to join you. Have each person submit a motivation—a quote from pop culture, literature, or history that captures their fitness goals and introduces them as the leader. You can email one another or set up a private Facebook group. Send exercise challenges each week. Share articles and encouragement along the way. You will soon learn that each person finds his or her motivation in different ways. And having a change in leadership each month can uncover strengths and resources you didn't know existed. This is a great way to push beyond your personal limits and keep the positivity flowing all year long.

required, no time wasted on the commute, and no inclement weather barriers. The time flies! If you don't have a machine, you can stroll the neighborhood or the hallway, or take the stairs.

Connecting to Our Communities

Sometimes the responsibilities and routines of life take over and months or years can go by where we never venture beyond our own metaphorical front yards. And even if we do, how often do we really interact with people and experience cultures outside of our own? Get out of your routine once in a while. See what's happening right around where you live. What's going on in your area that matters to you? You don't have to run for city council to connect with the concerns in the place you call home. Attend a city council meeting, a ribbon-cutting ceremony, or a store opening. What about local museums, cultural festivals, or the elementary school rendition of *Annie*? It may not be Broadway, but it's your neighborhood.

Take a day trip sometime. Pick a town an hour or so away from where you live, grab a friend or go alone, play some really great music on the drive, and spend the day exploring and connecting to the people and the area. You don't need big, elaborate plans to be a tourist. Visit the town's tourist bureau, or talk to the locals and find the best places to see. Stroll along Main Street. Have lunch or dinner in a quaint restaurant.

These types of experiences don't have to require great effort, significant time or money, or a long-term commitment. They offer an element of surprise and curiosity that opens you up for more connection. You're not just in your own world anymore. You're out there, appreciating the people, places, and a good life!

Do Good, Feel Great

Do you care so much about a cause that you're willing to donate your time to make things better? If so, your compassion meter is running high. *Compassion* means "suffer together." When you witness a need in a vulnerable group, feel concerned for their welfare, and have the motivation to help, you're experiencing compassion. A step beyond empathy, feeling another's difficulty, compassion says, "I can do something about this." Audrey Hepburn said, "As you grow older you will discover you have two hands, one for helping yourself, the other for helping others."

Volunteering can truly change your perspective on your own situation and increase your sense of empathy for what other people may be going through. Through giving, we receive so much more than we could ever imagine, and often much more than we can even give. In helping others we are also helping ourselves and building our self-esteem. **Doing something for someone else activates the same part of our brain as treating ourselves well.** When an act of kindness is carried out, your brain associates this with pleasure, connection, and trust (an emotion on the level of love). And the bonus is that endorphins are released in all the people involved. Even witnessing another person's good deeds has a way of elevating us.

When I want a guaranteed "warm and fuzzy," all I have to do is think about my best friend, Dawn, and the love of her life, a dog named Monroe. Dawn volunteers with PetPromise, a no-kill animal welfare organization. Dawn refers to herself as a "foster failure" because she ended up adopting the very first dog she was supposed to house temporarily and help find a forever home. Over the years, Dawn has raised thousands of dollars and spent countless hours giving pets a better life. Home visits and vet checks for adoptions, approving and supporting foster families, and fostering puppies herself only scratch the surface of Dawn's dedication. She says, "Animals don't have a voice, so we need to speak for them. Dogs know they are being saved when I transport them from a kill shelter. They are so thankful, and I feel good being able to help." Rescuing Monroe has brought more happiness to Dawn's life than she ever imagined. They are best buddies, working out together, exploring nature, and cuddling on the sofa. Dawn's deep love for animals pulls her to do what she can to make a difference in their lives, and in return she feels appreciated and loved right back, in the form of puppy licks. Their special bond creates plenty of upward spirals in Dawn's life and certainly helps motivate her body kindness practice. But it would not exist if it weren't for Dawn's interest in being part of something more meaningful. What parts of your community compel you to get involved and make a difference?

Generosity has an interesting ripple effect. Originated from a single person, a generous act spreads by three degrees through a person's social network—from person to person, like a "kindness contagion." This means that each person in a network can influence dozens or even hundreds of people, including people you have never met! My upward spiral experience of receiving and sending flowers shows how one act can spark countless (often unknown) ripples of kindness.

When it comes to the transformative nature of community, no one knows better than award-winning author Glennon Doyle Melton. Through her popular online Momastery community and her brutally honest memoirs, *Carry*

On, Warrior and *Love Warrior*, Glennon shows up and shares every wonderful and ugly detail of her life, from struggling with alcoholism to an eating disorder to marriage difficulties. Despite getting sucker punched by life, she has healed herself and contributed to the healing of many people, earning the respect of Elizabeth Gilbert, Brené Brown, and others. Post by post, Glennon built a community of women who have "been there," connected by their shared experience and inspired to make things right. Asking, "How can I help?", Momastery's followers began planning local meetups and joined together to support other women online and in real life. The Momastery movement became truly official when Glennon and a group of its members founded the nonprofit organization Together Rising, which provides tangible ways for women across the world to connect and support one another. Whenever the site posts a need, community members rise to the occasion and send thousands of dollars for Haitian babies, blankets to refugees, or holiday gifts to struggling families in the US. Within hours the spirit of togetherness takes over and powerful things happen. Glennon calls on her community to practice "sistering"—women collaborating to strengthen one another by being there.

As human beings, our souls are desperate to find meaning and purpose beyond ourselves. The chance to connect with like-minded people and inspirational causes answers a longing deep within us. By joining together to support others we are honoring ourselves and acknowledging our common humanity and the responsibility of human beings to love all creatures. This is body kindness in the greatest sense of the word.

Connecting to Nature and the Planet

Whether it's a once-in-a-lifetime vacation or a day spent wandering on unfamiliar trails in your own hometown, we are drawn to connect with our world. When sparked, our senses of wonder and natural curiosity open our hearts and minds to the broader world outside of ourselves.

Taking the time to savor these moments keeps us connected to the past, present, and future, to humans and every living thing. You might have felt this if you have ever stared up at the majesty of a centuries-old redwood tree or out into the vastness of the Grand Canyon. For me, it's humbling to think of my own life in the context of such miraculous and historical beauty. How can I waste another moment of my short years on this planet downplaying the miracle of this body I have been given? From tiny cells we become the most beautiful thinking, breathing, feeling creatures on earth. What an amazing gift we have been given, and how dare we squander and abuse it?

How can you get away when a big vacation isn't in the cards? Take in

Spiral Up
GIVE YOURSELF SOME AWE

Wonder and awe are powerful positive emotions that we should all experience more often. One way to make this happen is to plan it. First, make a list of ten easy ways you can experience wonder and awe without leaving your town. You can probably even Google "best hiking trails in [insert city here]" or "top ten must-see places in [town]." Challenge yourself to discover someplace new within an hour's drive from your front door. Once you've covered all the unexpected adventures near home (you'll probably find some more along the way), make a bucket list of more distant, but doable, awe-inspiring adventures. Open up your calendar and schedule one.

nearby nature. Get soothed by the sun and waves from a nearby beach (if you're that lucky!). Feel the sand between your toes as you take a leisurely walk and search for seashells. Meander park paths, listening to the sounds of nature as you go. If there are grills at your park, plan a cookout. Sit beneath a tree, read a good book, or just nap. Any mountains close by? Drive along a scenic parkway. Hike the trails. Go leaf peeping in autumn. Deepening your connection to the world is often right at your doorstep. Getting outdoors and "going green" for a workout offers dual benefits, even if the weather isn't perfect. We should all spend at least fifteen minutes a day in sunshine to get our recommended dose of vitamin D (an important hormone for mood regulation and bone health). Walking is a sustainable activity. Every fifty thousand steps you take saves twenty-five car miles, over a gallon of gasoline. A little dose of nature naturally boosts your mood and makes you healthier. My mother-in-law is an avid hiker, and one of her rituals is the Japanese practice of *shinrin-yoku*, or forest bathing. Walking for a few hours mindfully in nature has been shown to reduce stress, anger, anxiety, and depression.

Your personal experiences with the wonder and awe that nature provides can set forth a cascade of life-changing events that can strengthen your health. For example, after being amazed at a beautiful sunset, maybe you get inspired to take better care of the planet. You might start in your home by recycling, conserving water, and reducing food waste. These goals can spark an interest in eating more plant-based foods, or learning more about the farm-to-table food movement. Perhaps you brush up on your meal planning creativity, so you buy less food to waste less food. Instead of calling for takeout, you decide to make a quick soup before your fresh food goes bad. Maybe you experiment with composting, join a CSA (Community Supported Agriculture) to get fresh food from regional farmers, or sign up for a community gardening plot. Maybe you start with a single potted basil plant on your kitchen windowsill. For some people, just keeping that plant alive will be enough to inspire wonder and awe! You might vow to buy fewer things that you don't really need, try to upcycle and create things you do need, or work with businesses that offer these items. Each time a new experience piques your curiosity, you can feel energized, interested, and excited about the ways that you are deepening your connection to the world.

When it comes to food and the environment, we are starting to become more aware of how our choices impact our planet. We hear about sustainability issues, see new products on the shelves, hear news stories, watch documentaries, and many people face a real challenge in deciding how to handle sustainability. Thoughts include "Should I go meat free?" and "But I can't afford organic milk!"—plus "Why are there so many options for eggs? Which one is the best?" Confusion can quickly escalate to anxiety, guilt, fear of judgment from others, and uncertainty. After exhausting themselves from overwhelming confusion, shoppers spiral downward in emotion, ultimately freezing them and leading them to inaction.

Sustainability offers a plethora of opportunities to practice body kindness for yourself and within your family, as well as opportunities to do good for the planet without necessarily following an unrealistic list of extreme rules. When someone asks me what to do, I say, "Do what is best for your family." There are always ways of making things work. I'll share what I do with my family in the hope of giving you ideas and inspiration to make your own path.

REDUCE FOOD WASTE IN MY HOME

Wasted food is the largest component of trash in the United States, making up 20 percent of landfills, where it produces methane gases that are even more potent in changing the climate than the often-discussed carbon dioxide. I do my part by planning, shopping, and preparing imperfect meals. I purchase only what I need, saving time and money.

BUY "UGLY" PRODUCE

Perfectly nutritious foods end up as grocery store waste. I'm lucky that the company Hungry Harvest is in my area. Operating like a CSA, Hungry Harvest delivers to my door a box of "ugly produce" that would otherwise go in landfills. For every box our family gets, Hungry Harvest also feeds a hungry family in our area. Besides feeling good about it, the produce delivery saves me time in the grocery store and provides an activity for me to do with my daughter. We use the produce we get as weekend cooking challenges. We still buy *pretty* produce too, of course. I have never found a CSA that fully met our family's desire for a variety of produce year-round. Even if you don't buy ugly produce you can always give away fresh food you can't use. AmpleHarvest.org helps gardeners donate extra produce to food pantries across America. Or inquire if you can drop good food off to a local organization in need.

COMPOST

We use a composting service that picks up our compostable food and paper product scraps each week. The company provides all the collection materials and delivers free bags of compost, which we use to grow a vegetable and herb garden in the summertime.

This investment is less than $50 a month, which we pull from our food and activities budget. We get to garden, cook, and eat together. I share these ideas not to suggest that these are things everyone should do, but to inspire you to

GROW IT YOURSELF

CONNECT THE EARTH WITH YOUR PLATE

INDOORS

Buy potted herbs, place them in a windowsill or nearby sunny spot, and use them in cooking.

Rosemary, basil, oregano, lavender, parsley, sage, chives, and mint can all thrive indoors.

OUTDOORS

Construct a garden box, build a raised garden bed, or plant directly into the ground. Choose a sunny spot with well-drained soil—at least six hours of full sun exposure and no puddles after a good rain.

Get familiar with edible crops and what they are like in terms of space, water, soil, and temperature.

Lettuces and other greens don't require much space or maintenance and grow quickly.

If your harvests taste good and make you feel good, you will feel more motivated to keep on growing. You can focus on plants that don't die easily, such as aloe, cactus, or geranium.

BONUS

People who use their green thumbs have less anxiety and lower blood pressure.

find ways you can feel good and do good that are particularly meaningful to you. Look up what you can do in your area or try other things that connect you to the planet, such as picking up litter or volunteering for an environmental cause. Everyone can make a difference in their own way without going to an extreme that stresses them out.

I'm reminded of the starfish parable. A man is walking along a beach where thousands of starfish are stranded in the sand, and he starts trying to help them get back to the water. Another man approaches, saying, "There are too many. You can't make a difference." The first man reaches down, picks up a starfish, throws it back in the ocean, and says, "I made a difference to that one." You do what you can, and the world is that much better for any tiny bit you can do. I wholeheartedly believe kindness to the planet matters, no matter where you live and how much time or money you have. Buy canned produce and recycle the cans. Ask people if they have extras from their CSA or garden that you can take off their hands. Make it a game to buy less and use what you buy. Everything you choose to do matters, and each choice has the ability to spiral upward beyond you. Sometimes you're planting a seed of kindness that won't fully develop until after you're gone. So today, in this moment, make choices that enhance your health, happiness, and body kindness practice, not take away from it.

Connecting to Spirit

Spirituality is a broad concept, based on the acceptance that all beings are connected to one another and to the planet. Often this includes belief in a greater power and a search for meaning and purpose in life. Your personal experiences with these connections—to self, others, nature, and the sacred—cannot be contrived. You might find comfort in art or nature, through service work, prayer, or practicing the ancient rituals of yoga and meditation.

For many people, a spiritual life is integrated with a church, mosque, temple, or synagogue. Increasingly, the overlap of religion and universal spirituality is becoming more evident. In Cleveland, Ohio, a group of Catholic nuns offers free, ancient Reiki energy treatments to the community, and it's not uncommon across the country to see a rabbi standing alongside a minister or priest performing interfaith celebrations or collaborating in social justice efforts.

For many reasons, spirituality is linked to happier, more fulfilling lives— which is the ultimate goal of practicing body kindness. People with a strong sense of spirituality are more likely to let go of their need to control outcomes. Realizing that you can't control situations can be a powerful discovery, with the potential to set you free from unnecessary suffering. Cultivating spirituality

Spiral Up
FIND YOUR SPIRITUAL SIDE

There will be a time when you're in search of peace, focus, energy, or self-love. Developing and practicing some rituals now will better prepare you to draw on them when you need them. Spend a few moments finding your favorite scriptures, poems, and quotes and put them all in one place. You could make your own book or keep a small collection in a sacred space in your house—a little nook by the window or a corner of your room. Put some yoga mantras set to music on your smartphone, or search for podcasts of a spiritual nature. Having a spiritual plan in place can be very reassuring. Aside from traditional religious teachings, consider reading about practices outside your own. Or keep a book of poems handy for times when you need a calming, spiritual shift. Rumi and Mary Oliver are great for this.

improves your emotional well-being as you experience big positive emotions like peace, awe, contentment, acceptance, empathy, and gratitude.

Leslie has felt the closeness of death more than enough for one lifetime. It began with her own complicated pregnancy and hospitalization over two months that nearly resulted in the loss of her baby and her own life. The trauma left her feeling raw, anxious, and alone, even though she had her "miracle baby" and plenty of people who loved her. Then a dear neighbor died. Then a close family member died. Both of those events hit her hard. And when her beloved friend Caroline was given two months to live at just thirty-eight years old, it was more than she could bear. An unusually harsh inner critic took over her mind with poisonous thoughts, such as, "You're a nobody. You're a terrible wife and mother." Leslie denied her depression and spiraled down for more than three years. Her hopelessness was so deep that her therapist, husband, or daughter couldn't seem to help. Leslie did not walk around with tear-filled swollen eyes, disheveled hair, and ratty pajamas. Her uniform was perfectly put together down to the glossy lipstick, but she was dying on the inside. Depression is most dangerous when it's well concealed. Leslie's drug was perfectionism. "If I could just launch this business product, I'd be more successful and everything would be fine."

But any emotional highs from business achievements quickly faded and she was left feeling hollow and worthless.

Then one day, as she numbly drove herself to work, she heard a song and woke up. "He Knows My Name" came on the radio, and Leslie remembered her faith and she began to think about God's faith in her. "Who am I to say I can't get out of this? Who am I to say I'm not good enough just as I am? God loves me, why can't I love me?" God had faith in her all along. She had just forgotten how to connect to it. Leslie realized that using business success to define her self-worth would never work for her. Lipstick was not going to solve her problems, but maybe faith would.

She prayed on this for a long time and she slowly began to spiral up. She took walks, began a prayer and gratitude journal, and eventually went back to her exercise class. She found the strength to be good to herself again through scripture, fellowship, therapy, and her family. Leslie knew that she would not let depression or anxiety rule her because she remembered the value of life—a life her dear young friend Caroline wanted so much for herself, but got cut short. Leslie committed to a new life plan in honor of her friend's memory—hug her child more, laugh every day, and be open to new experiences. In fact, Leslie took a big risk she never could have imagined a year prior. She agreed to sell her business and move her family to another state for her husband's career. They would all start over together, leaving a physical space behind and good memories in their hearts. **Leslie's spiritual connection saved her life.** Without her faith in God, Leslie believes she would still be lost and depressed, here but not really living. But when Leslie let herself be good enough, she was fully alive. And that woman was pretty damn good! She had her health, family, faith, and friends. What more did she really need? And no matter what the future holds, God will always love her and that's good enough for Leslie.

Who and what do you consider a part of your spiritual tribe? Spend a few minutes journaling about how your connections to a higher power, the energy of the universe, or nature can help you create a better life for yourself. Does spiritual connection help you to be kinder to yourself? What rituals, meditations, or spiritual exercises enhance your body kindness practice?

Connecting with the energy and kindness in your community and the world is always worth the time it takes to do. My friend Pam likes to say that "If you think the world is a terrible place, then you're just not spending enough time with the right people." Anything you can do to benefit others or be inspired will ultimately enhance the meaning and purpose of your own life. Be intentional about noticing and nurturing your web of connections. The same light that is hiding within you is inside each person you meet, just waiting to shine. It's time we start noticing it in ourselves, our families, and the world around us. One choice, one moment, one act of kindness at a time.

BODY KINDNESS REFLECTION: Spend a few minutes journaling about a community you would like to learn about or participate in. Reflect on what your ideal body kindness tribe may look like, one that enhances your goals and helps you create a better life.

Lokah Samastah
Sukhino Bhavantu

"May all beings be happy and free, and may all my thoughts, words, and actions contribute in some way to that happiness and to that freedom for all."

—Shanti mantra

What I've Learned

....

Body Kindness for Life

Coming Back to the
Heart of Body Kindness

You may have reached the end of the book, but this is not the end of your journey. Over the coming days and weeks, I encourage you to continue daily writing in your body kindness journal and look back to remind yourself of all your insights, dreams, and ideas. I hope your kind and loving inner caregiver is louder than it used to be and that you are listening and paying attention. If what you focus on becomes your life, then I want you to be able to say "life is good."

There may come a time when it feels like all your exciting body kindness work is a distant memory, and you start hearing that inner thought bully picking on you again. Just promise me one thing—that you will never think of yourself as a body kindness failure. Perfection has never been our goal. When the inevitable setbacks happen, it's time to reconnect with and strengthen your values. If things get tough, or you begin to question if you're going in the right direction, ask yourself the universal body kindness question: "Am I creating a better life for myself?" If you aren't choosing kindness, what one small thing can you do right now to change course and create an upward spiral?

Take as much time as you need to do this right. Pause. Break. Come back to it. Give yourself permission to stop and try again. Hit your "reset button" by asking what matters to you and why. Your "whys" may change over time. You have the rest of your life to get comfortable with the person you are becoming. Think of all the ways letting go has been part of the body kindness process—old unworkable habits, detaching from unhelpful feelings, changes in relationships, and belonging to a community that fits you.

But letting go is not easy. In a culture that says we should deprive ourselves, there's something very radical and rebellious about making truly satisfying choices and enjoying a life well-lived. Even as we finalized these pages for print, more scientific evidence was being published about the damaging effects of extreme weight loss strategies. I have little doubt that despite sensationalized headlines everywhere you look and click, science will continue to prove that health and weight are wrongly intertwined and that the value of real health is in developing a healthy well-being—a total mind and body wellness that cannot be defined by a number. My greatest wish is that someday this book will

Spiral Up

I f you could tell someone a short story about your beliefs on health and well-being, what would you say to them? Write your body kindness "story" in your journal. It doesn't need to be longer than one paragraph. If you summed up your body kindness story in just six words, what would your story say? How do you feel when you read it out loud?

become outdated because our culture has finally accepted a broader notion of what it means to be healthy, and being good to ourselves is a natural response.

I have hope that big change is coming. I saw it when plus-sized model and body activist Ashley Graham made the cover of *Sports Illustrated* Swimsuit edition and when the "new" Barbie started looking more like the shapes, colors, and sizes of real people I know. I see it when diet foods and weight loss programs continue to lose money hand over fist. But we have a long way to go in our society. I believe the greatest impact can be made by you looking in the mirror and saying, "I can make a difference." If thousands of us fully commit, it's bound to make waves. Maya Angelou famously said, "I did then what I knew how to do. Now that I know better, I do better." Let that become a guiding truth for the rest of us. We know better. We can do better. We *must* do better—for our sisters, friends, daughters, and for ourselves.

> "No act of kindness, no matter how small, is ever wasted."
>
> —Aesop

Five Things You Can Do to Spread Body Kindness to the World

1 Elevate your conversations to things more important than appearance. When given the chance, teach friends and family to make choices that help them create a better life.

2 Care about yourself enough to not care too much. Shake off judgments from others and yourself. When in doubt, come back to the body kindness pillars of love, connect, and care.

3 Be brave. Share body kindness with those you care about. Speak up and use your powerful, educated voice for good.

4 Vote with your dollar. Support communities and businesses that make room for everyone in their definition of health and beauty.

5 Build a strong tribe and share your kindness, gratitude, and passion for life with as many people as possible.

Acknowledgments

In a world full of "no," there were three essential "yes" women who made this book possible:

Carol Blymire, my publicist: Thank you for believing there was a book in me and for having all the confidence when I was full of uncertainty.

Anna Sproul-Latimer, my agent: Thank you for believing my book could change lives and for your unparalleled commitment to my success throughout this entire process.

Mary Ellen O'Neill, my editor: Thank you for believing the time was right for our culture to embrace a compassionate approach to health. You have been a true partner in every sense of the word.

To my Workman family: You are amazing! Thank you for all your efforts, seen and unseen, in putting this book into the hands of the people who need it most. I especially thank Suzie Bolotin, publisher, who has been an enthusiastic champion of this project from the beginning. Thank you to Jean-Marc Troadec for the beautiful interior design, and to Jean-Marc, Vaughn Andrews, and James Williamson for the lively infographics. Janet Vicario for finally nailing the cover! Kate Karol, Jessica Rozler, Claire McKean, and Evan Griffith for your keen attention to every last detail in bringing manuscript pages to book form. Many thanks to Selina Meere, Jessica Wiener, Chloe Puton, and Lauren Southard for your tireless work in marketing and publicity.

Sincere appreciation goes out to the people who bravely shared their personal stories in the hope that they may help others. I especially thank Dawn Marsh, Pam Turos, Maggie Bright, Emily Halle, Vonda Smith, Kate Volzer, Bernie Salazar, Robby Lamb, Paola Neme, Rolando Murillo, Danielle West, and storyteller/filmmaker Kerith Lemon.

Friends and family members were valuable sounding boards for my ideas. I needed every one of you, especially Alison Sacks, Loren Bockweg, and Susan Scritchfield. Thanks for your research assistance and for helping to keep my business and life in working order.

Many professional colleagues have inspired me as I toiled with defining the kind of helping professional I wanted to be, and I'm forever grateful. Special thanks to Marsha Hudnall, Evelyn Tribole, Ellie Krieger, and of course, my "P's" Wendy Jo Peterson and Leslie Schilling.

To my Health at Every Size tribe: Thank you for doing the difficult work, day in and day out. We know it's worth it. I have faith society will catch up with science and humanity.

Thanks to my mom, Linda, for encouraging me to seek out happiness in my career and life. I would not have allowed myself to figure out what I was meant to do without this wisdom. (I will always be your cheerleader.)

To my husband, Andy: "Wow, look at us now! Flowers in the window." You are there for every step, big and small, and I can't imagine any greater privilege than watching our flowers grow together.

Finally, I'd like to thank some of my greatest teachers, my mistakes, for reminding me that I am a human being and that I am deserving of love, compassion, and understanding—no matter what!

About the Author

Rebecca Scritchfield, MA, RDN, ACSM HFS, believes that *true* health is not dependent on one's weight or pants size. Through her mindfulness-based counseling business, Rebecca helps people create better lives without dieting by showing them how to make self-care choices that fit their values, interests, and goals. In addition to speaking, writing, and podcasting about body kindness, she has appeared in over 100 broadcast television, radio, print, and online interviews, including *NBC Nightly News,* CNN, Fox News, the *Today* show, the *Washington Post, O, The Oprah Magazine, Health, Shape, Fit Pregnancy, Women's Health,* and many others.

Rebecca is passionate about shifting the cultural attitudes of health away from appearance and toward the well-being of individuals, families, and our communities. Her belief in body kindness was forged out of her own journey from body-hatred to self-acceptance and countless frustrating experiences with clients who rejected standard weight-loss tactics as joyless and unworkable!

As cofounder of Dietitians for Body Confidence, Rebecca is leading the charge of registered dietitian nutritionists who bravely say, "I will help you take good care of the body you have now."

Rebecca has a master's degree in communications from the Johns Hopkins University and bachelor degrees in chemistry and nutrition. She lives in Washington, DC, with her husband and two daughters. Her websites are bodykindnessbook.com and RebeccaScritchfield.com.